FREE Study Skills DVD Offer

FREE Study Skills DVD Offer

Dear Customer,

Thank you f
purchased o

As a way of
Skills DVD th
ready for yo
test.

All that we a
our product.

To get your F
the subject li

- The n
- Your
- Your
  impre
  study
  highli
- Your f

If you have an

Thanks again!

Sincerely,

Jay Willis
Vice President
jay.willis@mo
1-800-673-81

FREE Study Skills DVD Offer

Dear Customer,

Thank you for your purchase from Mometrix! We consider it an honor and privilege that you have purchased our product and want to ensure your satisfaction.

As a way of showing our appreciation and to help us better serve you, we have developed a Study Skills DVD that we would like to give you for FREE. **This DVD covers our "best practices" for studying for your exam, from using our study materials to preparing for the day of the test.**

All that we ask is that you email us your feedback that would describe your experience so far with our product. Good, bad or indifferent, we want to know what you think!

To get your **FREE Study Skills DVD**, email freedvd@mometrix.com with "FREE STUDY SKILLS DVD" in the subject line and the following information in the body of the email:

a. The name of the product you purchased.
b. Your product rating on a scale of 1-5, with 5 being the highest rating.
c. Your feedback. It can be long, short, or anything in-between, just your impressions and experience so far with our product. Good feedback might include how our study material met your needs and will highlight features of the product that you found helpful.
d. Your full name and shipping address where you would like us to send your free DVD.

If you have any questions or concerns, please don't hesitate to contact me directly. Thanks again!

Sincerely,

Jay Willis
Vice President
jay.willis@mometrix.com
1-800-673-8175

CHES
Exam
SECRETS

Study Guide
Your Key to Exam Success

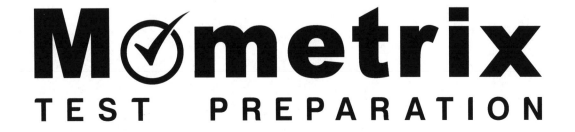

Written and edited by the Mometrix Health Educator Certification Test Team

Printed in the United States of America

This paper meets the requirements of ANSI/NISO Z39.48-1992 (Permanence of Paper).

Mometrix offers volume discount pricing to institutions. For more information or a price quote, please contact our sales department at sales@mometrix.com or 888-248-1219.

Paperback
ISBN 13: 978-1-60971-334-8
ISBN 10: 1-60971-334-6

Ebook
ISBN 13: 978-1-62120-504-3
ISBN 10: 1-62120-504-5

Dear Future Exam Success Story

First of all, **THANK YOU** for purchasing Mometrix study materials!

Second, congratulations! You are one of the few determined test-takers who are committed to doing whatever it takes to excel on your exam. **You have come to the right place.** We developed these study materials with one goal in mind: to deliver you the information you need in a format that's concise and easy to use.

In addition to optimizing your guide for the content of the test, we've outlined our recommended steps for breaking down the preparation process into small, attainable goals so you can make sure you stay on track.

We've also analyzed the entire test-taking process, identifying the most common pitfalls and showing how you can overcome them and be ready for any curveball the test throws you.

Standardized testing is one of the biggest obstacles on your road to success, which only increases the importance of doing well in the high-pressure, high-stakes environment of test day. Your results on this test could have a significant impact on your future, and this guide provides the information and practical advice to help you achieve your full potential on test day.

Your success is our success

We would love to hear from you! If you would like to share the story of your exam success or if you have any questions or comments in regard to our products, please contact us at **800-673-8175** or **support@mometrix.com**.

Thanks again for your business and we wish you continued success!

Sincerely,
The Mometrix Test Preparation Team

Need more help? Check out our flashcards at:
http://MometrixFlashcards.com/CHES

TABLE OF CONTENTS

Introduction

Thank you for purchasing this resource! You have made the choice to prepare yourself for a test that could have a huge impact on your future, and this guide is designed to help you be fully ready for test day. Obviously, it's important to have a solid understanding of the test material, but you also need to be prepared for the unique environment and stressors of the test, so that you can perform to the best of your abilities.

For this purpose, the first section that appears in this guide is the **Secret Keys**. We've devoted countless hours to meticulously researching what works and what doesn't, and we've boiled down our findings to the five most impactful steps you can take to improve your performance on the test. We start at the beginning with study planning and move through the preparation process, all the way to the testing strategies that will help you get the most out of what you know when you're finally sitting in front of the test.

We recommend that you start preparing for your test as far in advance as possible. However, if you've bought this guide as a last-minute study resource and only have a few days before your test, we recommend that you skip over the first two Secret Keys since they address a long-term study plan.

If you struggle with **test anxiety**, we strongly encourage you to check out our recommendations for how you can overcome it. Test anxiety is a formidable foe, but it can be beaten, and we want to make sure you have the tools you need to defeat it.

Secret Key #1 – Plan Big, Study Small

There's a lot riding on your performance. If you want to ace this test, you're going to need to keep your skills sharp and the material fresh in your mind. You need a plan that lets you review everything you need to know while still fitting in your schedule. We'll break this strategy down into three categories.

Information Organization

Start with the information you already have: the official test outline. From this, you can make a complete list of all the concepts you need to cover before the test. Organize these concepts into groups that can be studied together, and create a list of any related vocabulary you need to learn so you can brush up on any difficult terms. You'll want to keep this vocabulary list handy once you actually start studying since you may need to add to it along the way.

Time Management

Once you have your set of study concepts, decide how to spread them out over the time you have left before the test. Break your study plan into small, clear goals so you have a manageable task for each day and know exactly what you're doing. Then just focus on one small step at a time. When you manage your time this way, you don't need to spend hours at a time studying. Studying a small block of content for a short period each day helps you retain information better and avoid stressing over how much you have left to do. You can relax knowing that you have a plan to cover everything in time. In order for this strategy to be effective though, you have to start studying early and stick to your schedule. Avoid the exhaustion and futility that comes from last-minute cramming!

Study Environment

The environment you study in has a big impact on your learning. Studying in a coffee shop, while probably more enjoyable, is not likely to be as fruitful as studying in a quiet room. It's important to keep distractions to a minimum. You're only planning to study for a short block of time, so make the most of it. Don't pause to check your phone or get up to find a snack. It's also important to **avoid multitasking**. Research has consistently shown that multitasking will make your studying dramatically less effective. Your study area should also be comfortable and well-lit so you don't have the distraction of straining your eyes or sitting on an uncomfortable chair.

The time of day you study is also important. You want to be rested and alert. Don't wait until just before bedtime. Study when you'll be most likely to comprehend and remember. Even better, if you know what time of day your test will be, set that time aside for study. That way your brain will be used to working on that subject at that specific time and you'll have a better chance of recalling information.

Finally, it can be helpful to team up with others who are studying for the same test. Your actual studying should be done in as isolated an environment as possible, but the work of organizing the information and setting up the study plan can be divided up. In between study sessions, you can discuss with your teammates the concepts that you're all studying and quiz each other on the details. Just be sure that your teammates are as serious about the test as you are. If you find that your study time is being replaced with social time, you might need to find a new team.

Secret Key #2 – Make Your Studying Count

You're devoting a lot of time and effort to preparing for this test, so you want to be absolutely certain it will pay off. This means doing more than just reading the content and hoping you can remember it on test day. It's important to make every minute of study count. There are two main areas you can focus on to make your studying count:

Retention

It doesn't matter how much time you study if you can't remember the material. You need to make sure you are retaining the concepts. To check your retention of the information you're learning, try recalling it at later times with minimal prompting. Try carrying around flashcards and glance at one or two from time to time or ask a friend who's also studying for the test to quiz you.

To enhance your retention, look for ways to put the information into practice so that you can apply it rather than simply recalling it. If you're using the information in practical ways, it will be much easier to remember. Similarly, it helps to solidify a concept in your mind if you're not only reading it to yourself but also explaining it to someone else. Ask a friend to let you teach them about a concept you're a little shaky on (or speak aloud to an imaginary audience if necessary). As you try to summarize, define, give examples, and answer your friend's questions, you'll understand the concepts better and they will stay with you longer. Finally, step back for a big picture view and ask yourself how each piece of information fits with the whole subject. When you link the different concepts together and see them working together as a whole, it's easier to remember the individual components.

Finally, practice showing your work on any multi-step problems, even if you're just studying. Writing out each step you take to solve a problem will help solidify the process in your mind, and you'll be more likely to remember it during the test.

Modality

Modality simply refers to the means or method by which you study. Choosing a study modality that fits your own individual learning style is crucial. No two people learn best in exactly the same way, so it's important to know your strengths and use them to your advantage.

For example, if you learn best by visualization, focus on visualizing a concept in your mind and draw an image or a diagram. Try color-coding your notes, illustrating them, or creating symbols that will trigger your mind to recall a learned concept. If you learn best by hearing or discussing information, find a study partner who learns the same way or read aloud to yourself. Think about how to put the information in your own words. Imagine that you are giving a lecture on the topic and record yourself so you can listen to it later.

For any learning style, flashcards can be helpful. Organize the information so you can take advantage of spare moments to review. Underline key words or phrases. Use different colors for different categories. Mnemonic devices (such as creating a short list in which every item starts with the same letter) can also help with retention. Find what works best for you and use it to store the information in your mind most effectively and easily.

3

Secret Key #3 – Practice the Right Way

Your success on test day depends not only on how many hours you put into preparing, but also on whether you prepared the right way. It's good to check along the way to see if your studying is paying off. One of the most effective ways to do this is by taking practice tests to evaluate your progress. Practice tests are useful because they show exactly where you need to improve. Every time you take a practice test, pay special attention to these three groups of questions:

- The questions you got wrong
- The questions you had to guess on, even if you guessed right
- The questions you found difficult or slow to work through

This will show you exactly what your weak areas are, and where you need to devote more study time. Ask yourself why each of these questions gave you trouble. Was it because you didn't understand the material? Was it because you didn't remember the vocabulary? Do you need more repetitions on this type of question to build speed and confidence? Dig into those questions and figure out how you can strengthen your weak areas as you go back to review the material.

Additionally, many practice tests have a section explaining the answer choices. It can be tempting to read the explanation and think that you now have a good understanding of the concept. However, an explanation likely only covers part of the question's broader context. Even if the explanation makes sense, **go back and investigate** every concept related to the question until you're positive you have a thorough understanding.

As you go along, keep in mind that the practice test is just that: practice. Memorizing these questions and answers will not be very helpful on the actual test because it is unlikely to have any of the same exact questions. If you only know the right answers to the sample questions, you won't be prepared for the real thing. **Study the concepts** until you understand them fully, and then you'll be able to answer any question that shows up on the test.

It's important to wait on the practice tests until you're ready. If you take a test on your first day of study, you may be overwhelmed by the amount of material covered and how much you need to learn. Work up to it gradually.

On test day, you'll need to be prepared for answering questions, managing your time, and using the test-taking strategies you've learned. It's a lot to balance, like a mental marathon that will have a big impact on your future. Like training for a marathon, you'll need to start slowly and work your way up. When test day arrives, you'll be ready.

Start with the strategies you've read in the first two Secret Keys—plan your course and study in the way that works best for you. If you have time, consider using multiple study resources to get different approaches to the same concepts. It can be helpful to see difficult concepts from more than one angle. Then find a good source for practice tests. Many times, the test website will suggest potential study resources or provide sample tests.

Practice Test Strategy

When you're ready to start taking practice tests, follow this strategy:

UNTIMED AND OPEN-BOOK PRACTICE

Take the first test with no time constraints and with your notes and study guide handy. Take your time and focus on applying the strategies you've learned.

TIMED AND OPEN-BOOK PRACTICE

Take the second practice test open-book as well, but set a timer and practice pacing yourself to finish in time.

TIMED AND CLOSED-BOOK PRACTICE

Take any other practice tests as if it were test day. Set a timer and put away your study materials. Sit at a table or desk in a quiet room, imagine yourself at the testing center, and answer questions as quickly and accurately as possible.

Keep repeating timed and closed-book tests on a regular basis until you run out of practice tests or it's time for the actual test. Your mind will be ready for the schedule and stress of test day, and you'll be able to focus on recalling the material you've learned.

Secret Key #4 – Pace Yourself

Once you're fully prepared for the material on the test, your biggest challenge on test day will be managing your time. Just knowing that the clock is ticking can make you panic even if you have plenty of time left. Work on pacing yourself so you can build confidence against the time constraints of the exam. Pacing is a difficult skill to master, especially in a high-pressure environment, so **practice is vital**.

Set time expectations for your pace based on how much time is available. For example, if a section has 60 questions and the time limit is 30 minutes, you know you have to average 30 seconds or less per question in order to answer them all. Although 30 seconds is the hard limit, set 25 seconds per question as your goal, so you reserve extra time to spend on harder questions. When you budget extra time for the harder questions, you no longer have any reason to stress when those questions take longer to answer.

Don't let this time expectation distract you from working through the test at a calm, steady pace, but keep it in mind so you don't spend too much time on any one question. Recognize that taking extra time on one question you don't understand may keep you from answering two that you do understand later in the test. If your time limit for a question is up and you're still not sure of the answer, mark it and move on, and come back to it later if the time and the test format allow. If the testing format doesn't allow you to return to earlier questions, just make an educated guess; then put it out of your mind and move on.

On the easier questions, be careful not to rush. It may seem wise to hurry through them so you have more time for the challenging ones, but it's not worth missing one if you know the concept and just didn't take the time to read the question fully. Work efficiently but make sure you understand the question and have looked at all of the answer choices, since more than one may seem right at first.

Even if you're paying attention to the time, you may find yourself a little behind at some point. You should speed up to get back on track, but do so wisely. Don't panic; just take a few seconds less on each question until you're caught up. Don't guess without thinking, but do look through the answer choices and eliminate any you know are wrong. If you can get down to two choices, it is often worthwhile to guess from those. Once you've chosen an answer, move on and don't dwell on any that you skipped or had to hurry through. If a question was taking too long, chances are it was one of the harder ones, so you weren't as likely to get it right anyway.

On the other hand, if you find yourself getting ahead of schedule, it may be beneficial to slow down a little. The more quickly you work, the more likely you are to make a careless mistake that will affect your score. You've budgeted time for each question, so don't be afraid to spend that time. Practice an efficient but careful pace to get the most out of the time you have.

Secret Key #5 – Have a Plan for Guessing

When you're taking the test, you may find yourself stuck on a question. Some of the answer choices seem better than others, but you don't see the one answer choice that is obviously correct. What do you do?

The scenario described above is very common, yet most test takers have not effectively prepared for it. Developing and practicing a plan for guessing may be one of the single most effective uses of your time as you get ready for the exam.

In developing your plan for guessing, there are three questions to address:

- When should you start the guessing process?
- How should you narrow down the choices?
- Which answer should you choose?

When to Start the Guessing Process

Unless your plan for guessing is to select C every time (which, despite its merits, is not what we recommend), you need to leave yourself enough time to apply your answer elimination strategies. Since you have a limited amount of time for each question, that means that if you're going to give yourself the best shot at guessing correctly, you have to decide quickly whether or not you will guess.

Of course, the best-case scenario is that you don't have to guess at all, so first, see if you can answer the question based on your knowledge of the subject and basic reasoning skills. Focus on the key words in the question and try to jog your memory of related topics. Give yourself a chance to bring the knowledge to mind, but once you realize that you don't have (or you can't access) the knowledge you need to answer the question, it's time to start the guessing process.

It's almost always better to start the guessing process too early than too late. It only takes a few seconds to remember something and answer the question from knowledge. Carefully eliminating wrong answer choices takes longer. Plus, going through the process of eliminating answer choices can actually help jog your memory.

Summary: Start the guessing process as soon as you decide that you can't answer the question based on your knowledge.

How to Narrow Down the Choices

The next chapter in this book (**Test-Taking Strategies**) includes a wide range of strategies for how to approach questions and how to look for answer choices to eliminate. You will definitely want to read those carefully, practice them, and figure out which ones work best for you. Here though, we're going to address a mindset rather than a particular strategy.

Your chances of guessing an answer correctly depend on how many options you are choosing from.

How many choices you have	How likely you are to guess correctly
5	20%
4	25%
3	33%
2	50%
1	100%

You can see from this chart just how valuable it is to be able to eliminate incorrect answers and make an educated guess, but there are two things that many test takers do that cause them to miss out on the benefits of guessing:

- Accidentally eliminating the correct answer
- Selecting an answer based on an impression

We'll look at the first one here, and the second one in the next section.

To avoid accidentally eliminating the correct answer, we recommend a thought exercise called **the $5 challenge**. In this challenge, you only eliminate an answer choice from contention if you are willing to bet $5 on it being wrong. Why $5? Five dollars is a small but not insignificant amount of money. It's an amount you could afford to lose but wouldn't want to throw away. And while losing $5 once might not hurt too much, doing it twenty times will set you back $100. In the same way, each small decision you make—eliminating a choice here, guessing on a question there—won't by itself impact your score very much, but when you put them all together, they can make a big difference. By holding each answer choice elimination decision to a higher standard, you can reduce the risk of accidentally eliminating the correct answer.

The $5 challenge can also be applied in a positive sense: If you are willing to bet $5 that an answer choice *is* correct, go ahead and mark it as correct.

Summary: Only eliminate an answer choice if you are willing to bet $5 that it is wrong.

Which Answer to Choose

You're taking the test. You've run into a hard question and decided you'll have to guess. You've eliminated all the answer choices you're willing to bet $5 on. Now you have to pick an answer. Why do we even need to talk about this? Why can't you just pick whichever one you feel like when the time comes?

The answer to these questions is that if you don't come into the test with a plan, you'll rely on your impression to select an answer choice, and if you do that, you risk falling into a trap. The test writers know that everyone who takes their test will be guessing on some of the questions, so they intentionally write wrong answer choices to seem plausible. You still have to pick an answer though, and if the wrong answer choices are designed to look right, how can you ever be sure that you're not falling for their trap? The best solution we've found to this dilemma is to take the decision out of your hands entirely. Here is the process we recommend:

Once you've eliminated any choices that you are confident (willing to bet $5) are wrong, select the first remaining choice as your answer.

Whether you choose to select the first remaining choice, the second, or the last, the important thing is that you use some preselected standard. Using this approach guarantees that you will not be enticed into selecting an answer choice that looks right, because you are not basing your decision on how the answer choices look.

This is not meant to make you question your knowledge. Instead, it is to help you recognize the difference between your knowledge and your impressions. There's a huge difference between thinking an answer is right because of what you know, and thinking an answer is right because it looks or sounds like it should be right.

Summary: To ensure that your selection is appropriately random, make a predetermined selection from among all answer choices you have not eliminated.

Test-Taking Strategies

This section contains a list of test-taking strategies that you may find helpful as you work through the test. By taking what you know and applying logical thought, you can maximize your chances of answering any question correctly!

It is very important to realize that every question is different and every person is different: no single strategy will work on every question, and no single strategy will work for every person. That's why we've included all of them here, so you can try them out and determine which ones work best for different types of questions and which ones work best for you.

Question Strategies

READ CAREFULLY

Read the question and answer choices carefully. Don't miss the question because you misread the terms. You have plenty of time to read each question thoroughly and make sure you understand what is being asked. Yet a happy medium must be attained, so don't waste too much time. You must read carefully, but efficiently.

CONTEXTUAL CLUES

Look for contextual clues. If the question includes a word you are not familiar with, look at the immediate context for some indication of what the word might mean. Contextual clues can often give you all the information you need to decipher the meaning of an unfamiliar word. Even if you can't determine the meaning, you may be able to narrow down the possibilities enough to make a solid guess at the answer to the question.

PREFIXES

If you're having trouble with a word in the question or answer choices, try dissecting it. Take advantage of every clue that the word might include. Prefixes and suffixes can be a huge help. Usually they allow you to determine a basic meaning. Pre- means before, post- means after, pro - is positive, de- is negative. From prefixes and suffixes, you can get an idea of the general meaning of the word and try to put it into context.

HEDGE WORDS

Watch out for critical hedge words, such as *likely, may, can, sometimes, often, almost, mostly, usually, generally, rarely,* and *sometimes.* Question writers insert these hedge phrases to cover every possibility. Often an answer choice will be wrong simply because it leaves no room for exception. Be on guard for answer choices that have definitive words such as *exactly* and *always.*

SWITCHBACK WORDS

Stay alert for *switchbacks.* These are the words and phrases frequently used to alert you to shifts in thought. The most common switchback words are *but, although,* and *however.* Others include *nevertheless, on the other hand, even though, while, in spite of, despite, regardless of.* Switchback words are important to catch because they can change the direction of the question or an answer choice.

FACE VALUE

When in doubt, use common sense. Accept the situation in the problem at face value. Don't read too much into it. These problems will not require you to make wild assumptions. If you have to go beyond creativity and warp time or space in order to have an answer choice fit the question, then you should move on and consider the other answer choices. These are normal problems rooted in reality. The applicable relationship or explanation may not be readily apparent, but it is there for you to figure out. Use your common sense to interpret anything that isn't clear.

Answer Choice Strategies

ANSWER SELECTION

The most thorough way to pick an answer choice is to identify and eliminate wrong answers until only one is left, then confirm it is the correct answer. Sometimes an answer choice may immediately seem right, but be careful. The test writers will usually put more than one reasonable answer choice on each question, so take a second to read all of them and make sure that the other choices are not equally obvious. As long as you have time left, it is better to read every answer choice than to pick the first one that looks right without checking the others.

ANSWER CHOICE FAMILIES

An answer choice family consists of two (in rare cases, three) answer choices that are very similar in construction and cannot all be true at the same time. If you see two answer choices that are direct opposites or parallels, one of them is usually the correct answer. For instance, if one answer choice says that quantity x increases and another either says that quantity x decreases (opposite) or says that quantity y increases (parallel), then those answer choices would fall into the same family. An answer choice that doesn't match the construction of the answer choice family is more likely to be incorrect. Most questions will not have answer choice families, but when they do appear, you should be prepared to recognize them.

ELIMINATE ANSWERS

Eliminate answer choices as soon as you realize they are wrong, but make sure you consider all possibilities. If you are eliminating answer choices and realize that the last one you are left with is also wrong, don't panic. Start over and consider each choice again. There may be something you missed the first time that you will realize on the second pass.

AVOID FACT TRAPS

Don't be distracted by an answer choice that is factually true but doesn't answer the question. You are looking for the choice that answers the question. Stay focused on what the question is asking for so you don't accidentally pick an answer that is true but incorrect. Always go back to the question and make sure the answer choice you've selected actually answers the question and is not merely a true statement.

EXTREME STATEMENTS

In general, you should avoid answers that put forth extreme actions as standard practice or proclaim controversial ideas as established fact. An answer choice that states the "process should be used in certain situations, if..." is much more likely to be correct than one that states the "process should be discontinued completely." The first is a calm rational statement and doesn't even make a definitive, uncompromising stance, using a hedge word *if* to provide wiggle room, whereas the second choice is a radical idea and far more extreme.

11

BENCHMARK

As you read through the answer choices and you come across one that seems to answer the question well, mentally select that answer choice. This is not your final answer, but it's the one that will help you evaluate the other answer choices. The one that you selected is your benchmark or standard for judging each of the other answer choices. Every other answer choice must be compared to your benchmark. That choice is correct until proven otherwise by another answer choice beating it. If you find a better answer, then that one becomes your new benchmark. Once you've decided that no other choice answers the question as well as your benchmark, you have your final answer.

PREDICT THE ANSWER

Before you even start looking at the answer choices, it is often best to try to predict the answer. When you come up with the answer on your own, it is easier to avoid distractions and traps because you will know exactly what to look for. The right answer choice is unlikely to be word-for-word what you came up with, but it should be a close match. Even if you are confident that you have the right answer, you should still take the time to read each option before moving on.

General Strategies

TOUGH QUESTIONS

If you are stumped on a problem or it appears too hard or too difficult, don't waste time. Move on! Remember though, if you can quickly check for obviously incorrect answer choices, your chances of guessing correctly are greatly improved. Before you completely give up, at least try to knock out a couple of possible answers. Eliminate what you can and then guess at the remaining answer choices before moving on.

CHECK YOUR WORK

Since you will probably not know every term listed and the answer to every question, it is important that you get credit for the ones that you do know. Don't miss any questions through careless mistakes. If at all possible, try to take a second to look back over your answer selection and make sure you've selected the correct answer choice and haven't made a costly careless mistake (such as marking an answer choice that you didn't mean to mark). This quick double check should more than pay for itself in caught mistakes for the time it costs.

PACE YOURSELF

It's easy to be overwhelmed when you're looking at a page full of questions; your mind is confused and full of random thoughts, and the clock is ticking down faster than you would like. Calm down and maintain the pace that you have set for yourself. Especially as you get down to the last few minutes of the test, don't let the small numbers on the clock make you panic. As long as you are on track by monitoring your pace, you are guaranteed to have time for each question.

DON'T RUSH

It is very easy to make errors when you are in a hurry. Maintaining a fast pace in answering questions is pointless if it makes you miss questions that you would have gotten right otherwise. Test writers like to include distracting information and wrong answers that seem right. Taking a little extra time to avoid careless mistakes can make all the difference in your test score. Find a pace that allows you to be confident in the answers that you select.

KEEP MOVING

Panicking will not help you pass the test, so do your best to stay calm and keep moving. Taking deep breaths and going through the answer elimination steps you practiced can help to break through a stress barrier and keep your pace.

Final Notes

The combination of a solid foundation of content knowledge and the confidence that comes from practicing your plan for applying that knowledge is the key to maximizing your performance on test day. As your foundation of content knowledge is built up and strengthened, you'll find that the strategies included in this chapter become more and more effective in helping you quickly sift through the distractions and traps of the test to isolate the correct answer.

Now it's time to move on to the test content chapters of this book, but be sure to keep your goal in mind. As you read, think about how you will be able to apply this information on the test. If you've already seen sample questions for the test and you have an idea of the question format and style, try to come up with questions of your own that you can answer based on what you're reading. This will give you valuable practice applying your knowledge in the same ways you can expect to on test day.

Good luck and good studying!

14

Assess Needs, Resources, and Capacity for Health Education/Promotion

ASSESSING A COMMUNITY'S NEED FOR HEALTH EDUCATION

Health educators need to go through a series of steps while determining what health programs would be most effective in a given community. To begin with, they will need to survey the available primary and secondary data. This should give an indication of what health problems are most pertinent in the community, as well as the various means by which these problems may be resolved. The health educator will also need to conduct a needs assessment and resource inventory at this point, in part to determine how much money, manpower, and community support he or she can count on for the program.

NEEDS ASSESSMENT

Needs assessments are performed to obtain health information about an individual or group. They are performed for a variety of different reasons and may include a number of different pieces of information. Most needs assessments, however, will include the following: the individual or group's current knowledge of health; the individual or group's attitude towards health; recommendations for health education; and any relevant socio-economic practices. The basic point of any needs assessment is to determine what kind of health education would be most beneficial for a given individual or community. In some cases, a needs assessment may indicate that individuals are in need of basics like food and shelter. Other needs assessments may indicate that a particular individual or community is susceptible to a specific physical or emotional problem.

Terms relative to a needs assessment:

- Community analysis: The process of assembling information about the target individual, group, or community; includes general health summary and evaluation of available health care
- Community diagnosis: Professional opinion of the health of the individual or community based on community analysis; special consideration to health problems as they relate to available health services
- Primary data: All the information collected directly by the health professional from the target individual, group, or community
- Secondary data: Any pertinent information not collected directly by the health professional

ETHICAL ISSUES

Ethical issues should always be considered during the process of assessment for health education. The people being assessed should understand the purpose of assessment, the method of assessment, the scoring method, and the assessment conditions. Informed consent is essential as well as feedback to the participants about the results of the assessment and access to data. The health education specialist should use up-to-date assessment methods that have both reliability and validity and should be trained to carry out the specific type of assessment. The assessment instrument used must be valid for the intended purpose. The health education specialist or person who directs the assessment is responsible for the assessment and dealing with the results even if the scoring is done automatically (such as through online testing) and must make sure that no harm comes to participants because of the assessment process. Security of the data and confidentiality must be assured.

15

Methods of Assessment and Analyzing Assessment Findings

The PRECEDE-PROCEED model utilizes the following assessments to establish needs for health education: social assessment, epidemiological assessment, behavioral and environmental assessment, educational and ecological assessment, and administrative and policy assessment. The social assessment measures the perception of the target population's quality of life and aids in the identification of the social conditions that will benefit from health education. The epidemiological assessment identifies the health issues exhibited by the target population and the behaviors and risks associated with said health problems; it also enables a baseline to be set for health educational priorities.

Computerized Information Sources

Thankfully, there are a bunch of helpful sources of data on health-related issues at present. These resources are invaluable minds of information for health educators. They are available through most university libraries and indeed through some public libraries as well. Some databases require a small membership fee. At present, some of the more popular databases are the Behavioral Risk Factor Surveillance System, the Education Resources Information Center, and the database PubMed operated by the National Library of Medicine.

Databases

There are number of ways in which databases may be useful in accessing health-related data. Most towns and communities keep extensive records of health-related issues, which educators can mine for clues about which problems affect a population the most, as well as how these problems may be resolved. Even better, much of this data is now housed on the Internet, which makes access all the easier. One problem that educators may have now, and which rarely occurred in the past, is an overabundance of information. For this reason, it is important to only use the information that most directly applies to the given situation.

Selecting Educational Information

A health educator is often referred to as a "clearinghouse" of information because he or she is responsible for selecting appropriate health-related resources to be distributed in a community. Furthermore, a health educator has to be able to select the right educational information sources for making decisions about program planning and implementation. In order to do this effectively, a health educator needs to stay abreast of all the various sources for health information. Medical and sociological research is constantly improving our understanding of basic health problems; health educators need to be able to find the most important sources of this new information.

Primary Data

Primary data is data that is obtained by the health education specialist via survey, interview, focus group, or direct observation of the focused person or population. Secondary data is established data that may or may not be concerning the focused person or population; examples include Vital Records, Disease Registry, U. S. Census, etc. There are multiple models used to identify gaps in data or to collect data to establish needs assessments. Such models are the epidemiological model, public health model, social model, asset model, and rapid model. Public computerized data bases may also be used.

Methods of gathering primary data:

- Resource inventories: Interviews are performed and records are scrutinized to determine which health services are being administered in a target community; a resource inventory depends on the accuracy of records

16

- Observation: Health professional watches target individual or community to obtain information; the health professional must be trained to keep accurate records
- Health Risk Appraisals/Assessments: A health professional uses the results of interviews and the analysis of records to determine an individual's long-term prognosis; specific factors like blood pressure and medical history are compared to sets of data to make an accurate prediction

SECONDARY DATA

In health education, secondary data is all of the information gathered about a subject that is not assembled through direct observation. In other words, secondary data includes all of the records maintained by other organizations, as for instance government agencies, state departments, and nonprofit organizations. As a health educator, you'll need to be able to seek out and extract appropriate information from secondary sources. Some of the common sources for secondary data are the Behavioral Risk Factor Surveillance System and the Youth Risk Behavior Surveillance System. Health educators also need to be familiar with sources of economic and demographic data.

Federal agencies that provide secondary data:

- National Center for Health Statistics: Assemblage of important health statistics
- Centers for Disease Control and Prevention (CDC): Compiles Morbidity and Mortality Weekly Report
- United States Department of Health and Human Services: Houses records of health programs and social assistance programs
- United States Census Bureau: Compiles various records all on population, socioeconomic class, education, and family size and composition; also publishes the invaluable Statistical Abstract of the United States

ESTABLISHING COLLABORATIVE RELATIONSHIPS THAT FACILITATE ACCESS TO DATA

Community organizing is very important in establishing collaborative relationships and agreements that facilitate access to data. Community organizing is defined as building an enduring network of people, who identify with common ideals, and who can engage in social action on the basis of those ideals. Community empowerment interventions are another important means in establishing collaborative relationships that facilitate data access. Community empowerment interventions serve to establish a wide change in health behaviors on a community level by creating organized communities that elaborate upon their health problems, determine the causes of their health problems, and subsequently work at appropriate individual and collective actions to alter such causes.

DETERMINING WHETHER DATA FROM DIFFERENT SOURCES IS COMPATIBLE

One problem which health educators currently face, which was never a problem before, is the possible overabundance of data. At times, a health educator may be overwhelmed by reams of data, making it almost impossible to interpret accurately. In order to minimize this problem, health educators should make sure to only use data from appropriate sources. Health educators should exclude any research data that is drawn from markedly different circumstances. Also, health educators should exclude any research that produces results wildly different than those of every other study; unless there is a solid explanation for these outlying results, it is safe to assume that they were produced by faulty research methods.

SURVEYS

In many cases, the information for a needs assessment can be assembled most easily by performing a survey. In order for the survey to be considered valid, the questions need to be specific and a large number of respondents need to be assembled. Health professionals will typically compare the results of a survey with previously-conducted surveys in order to ensure reliability. An effective survey must have a clear and appropriate objective, typically one that is established by all of those individuals with a direct interest in the results of the survey, known in the profession as stakeholders. The survey should be placed into terms that can be understood and responded to by a large number of individuals in the target community, so as to maximize the response rate. It is typical to combine the results of a survey with a recommended course of action.

Types of surveys:

- Mail surveys: One of the most common forms of survey; written surveys are sent through the mail to members of the target community; must be written in comprehensible language; responses are typically honest, but the response rate is low
- Telephone surveys: Inexpensive to perform and capable of assembling a great deal of information; obviously can only be performed on target population with telephones; high response rate, slightly less honesty than mail survey
- In-person (face-to-face) surveys: Often performed door to door; expensive to perform, but known for high response rate and attention to detail
- Interviews: Cost is proportionate to the number of people interviewed and the length of each interview; can derive detailed information if performed by a skilled interviewer

HEALTH NEEDS ASSESSMENTS

USING THE NOMINAL GROUP PROCESS TO GATHER DATA

Nominal groups are assembled when health professionals are specifically interested in developing a list of potential solutions to a health problem. In a nominal group, five to seven people are assembled and encouraged to rank a group of health issues in order of importance. This ranking may be preceded by a brief presentation on the health issues by a health professional. After the members of the group complete their hierarchy, they will be asked to brainstorm some possible solutions to the health problems they consider most important. A nominal group will be led by a facilitator, who is charged with completing the entire process within about an hour.

USING A COMMUNITY FORUM TO GATHER DATA

In a *community forum*, health professionals gather a number of representatives from the target community to discuss the health issue in question. Occasionally, a community forum will be initiated by a keynote speaker or presentation by a group of experts. Ideally, the representatives of the community will be from a variety of socioeconomic backgrounds. Community forms are good for getting the word out about important health issues, but are occasionally dominated by individuals with a particular ax to grind. Sometimes, marginal opinions may dominate the discussion to the detriment of the general audience.

USING FACE-TO-FACE SURVEYS TO GATHER INFORMATION

A *face-to-face survey* is only performed after the objectives of the survey have been clearly defined. A health professional must be well trained before undertaking a face-to-face survey. When performed correctly, this kind of survey can yield a huge amount of primary data. Also, a trained interviewer can ask subjects to elaborate on particular points to elicit helpful details. Of course,

18

face-to-face interviews only allow the researcher to obtain information from one individual at a time and are time consuming and expensive.

USING FOCUS GROUPS TO GATHER INFORMATION

Focus groups are specially-chosen collections of individuals brought together to answer questions and assess a presentation on a particular health issue. Focus groups are often initiated by some kind of visual presentation, led by a facilitator. After the presentation, the facilitator will help the group to discuss the health issue in question. Sometimes, other health professionals observe focus groups either through closed-circuit television or two-way mirrors. Because it can cost a fair amount of money to organize and conduct a focus group, the objectives of the survey must be explicit beforehand. Also, information obtained from the members of a focus group should not be extrapolated to apply to other individuals not represented by the focus group.

USING RESOURCE INVENTORIES TO GATHER INFORMATION

Resource inventories are performed to assess the availability and quality of health services in a particular community. In order to perform an accurate resource inventory, it is necessary to analyze the records of all pertinent agencies, perform interviews with local experts, and evaluate the strengths and weaknesses of the community healthcare. Of course, a resource inventory is only as accurate as the records that have been maintained; so, an important component of any resource inventory is an assessment of record quality and reliability.

USING A DELPHI PANEL TO GATHER INFORMATION

Health professionals usually perform a Delphi panel when it's impossible to gather all the individuals needed for a survey in the same place at the same time. A Delphi panel is performed as follows: questionnaires are sent out to each member of the group and the responses are analyzed by health professionals. The results of this analysis will determine subsequent questions. This process repeats itself through the course of three to five questionnaires. Most of the variations in Delphi panels have to do with sample size; the detailed and specific information obtained from targeted questionnaires enables a Delphi panel to be performed with a strikingly low number of participants.

RESPONSE RATES FOR MAIL SURVEYS VS. OTHER TYPES OF SURVEYS

Mail surveys have striking advantages and disadvantages. They are extremely inexpensive to perform and can be used to request information from a large group of people. Of course, as anyone who has received a mail survey can believe, there is a relatively low rate of response to this form of inquiry. Indeed, most mail surveys only have a response rate of between 5 and 10%. Phone surveys have a slightly higher response rate, but are more expensive. Door to door surveys have an even higher response rate, but are even more expensive.

DESIGNING AND COMPLETING A SURVEY

Before a survey can be designed and administered, specific objectives need to be defined. This is typically done in consultation with all of the stakeholders: those individuals who have a direct interest in the results of the study. It is only when the objective of the survey has been defined that the appropriate target population can be established. Once the target population has been identified, health professionals can discuss the specific data to be collected as well as the method for measuring it. At this point, health professionals will decide which form of survey is likely to yield the most appropriate data set. The survey can then be performed, after which point the results can be assessed for validity and reliability.

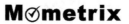

DATA COLLECTION PROCEDURES TO DETERMINE HEALTH EDUCATION NEEDS

When developing **data collection procedures** to determine health education needs, the health education specialist must consider the purpose of the data collection, the audience for which the data are intended, the types of questions to be answered, the scope of the research, and the resources available to carry out data collection:

Method	Issues regarding procedures
Direct observation	Observers must be selected and trained as to how to observe and when and how to record observations.
Interviews	Interview questions must be developed and validated and the interviewers given practice time.
Questionnaires	The type of questionnaire, the questions, and the Likert scale must be determined as well as the method of distribution (one-on-one, group, email, Internet).
Record review	A form or checklist should be developed to guide record review and the records selected based on criteria established for the research.
Secondary analysis	The databases to be mined should be selected and the criteria for the research established, including key words, timeframes, and populations.

TRAINING PERSONNEL TO ASSIST WITH DATA COLLECTION

When **training personnel** to assist with data collection, a number of topics must be covered:

- Purpose: The personnel should understand the purpose of the data collection.
- Method: The personnel should have step-by-step instructions and ample practice so that there is consistency in the method of collection because inconsistency can skew the results.
- Rights of those involved: The right to privacy and confidentiality, the right to agree to participate and to refuse should be clarified.
- Timeline: A timeline for collection should be established and reasonable goals set for collection during that period.
- Legal guidelines: Any legal issues should be outlined.
- Ethical issues: Discussion should include the Patient's Bill of Rights, the ANA Code of Ethics, and ethical principles (such as autonomy, beneficence, justice, and nonmalfeasance).
- Data storage: Personnel should have a clear understanding of how data is to be stored and secured, whether paper or electronic.

INTEGRATING PRIMARY AND SECONDARY DATA

There are many methods by which primary data are collected. These methods include interviews, surveys, focus groups, nominal group process, Delphi panels, observation, and self-assessments. Self-assessments have individuals complete questions regarding health history and create an assessment of risk when used in comparison to an established database. Delphi panels are a form of surveys in which those who participate may respond to the other ideas in the target population. A community analysis serves to collect primary data, and a community diagnosis will utilize the primary data and integrate it with secondary data.

BEHAVIORS THAT CAN IMPROVE OR WORSEN HEALTH IN A COMMUNITY

Even without realizing it, individuals can impact the health of their community by making positive or negative decisions. For instance, if the members of the community tend to be overweight, this will not encourage younger people to develop good eating habits and exercise routines. If,

20

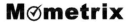

however, members of the community do develop healthy behaviors, these will likely spread to other individuals. Some of the health problems in a community will be the result of socioeconomic conditions, genetics, or the availability of health care, but others will be the direct result of the individual decisions made by the members of the community.

FACTORS INFLUENCING HEALTH BEHAVIORS

Health behaviors are a complex mix of *behavioral, environmental,* and *genetic factors.* The social health determinants include the following factors: early childhood development, education level, employment ability and type, food security, access to and quality of health care, living conditions and housing, income, discrimination, and social support. Biological factors including genetics, sex, and age impact health behavior. Health choices such as alcohol use, smoking, drug use, sexual activity, etc., also interact to influence health behaviors. Social characteristics, social environment, physical environment, and access to quality health care all contribute to health behaviors.

Genetic factors can have marked influence on health and health behaviors. Genetic factors serve to contribute to either a lesser or a greater risk for certain health outcomes as opposed to causing certain health outcomes definitively. There are links between genetic factors and behavior; studies of twins that were separated at birth show a high concordance rate of alcoholism, schizophrenia, and affective disorders (Baird, 1994). Some studies suggest that choice behaviors, such as smoking and diet, may be due to genetic factors. Social and environmental factors may interact with genetic factors to influence health behaviors.

FACTORS THAT ENHANCE OR COMPROMISE HEALTH

Genetic factors play a large role in either enhancing or compromising health. There are genetic predispositions for various disease states such as Alzheimer's disease, cardiovascular disease, diabetes, and stroke. Many forms of cancer can be genetic, and genetic testing may help in identifying genes associated with certain types of cancer. By knowing one's family history, one can take preventative measures to decrease the likelihood of developing such disease states, and thus enhance one's health. A strong genetic predisposition toward heart disease may allow an individual to alter his or her lifestyle in order to decrease the chances of sustaining heart attack or stroke.

Personal, economic, social, and *environmental elements* serve to either enhance or to compromise health. There are several categories of determinants of health. These categories include policy-making, social factors, health care services, individual behavior, and biology/genetics. Policy-making takes place at the local, state, and federal levels, and impacts individuals and entire communities and populations. Examples include steep tobacco taxes to decrease tobacco purchases and the 1966 Highway Safety Act and the National Traffic and Motor Vehicle Safety Act, which established standards and regulations for motor vehicles and roads.

INFLUENCE OF LIFESTYLE, ENVIRONMENTAL, AND INDIVIDUAL FACTORS ON HEALTHY BEHAVIOR

Health educators draw a distinction between behavioral, environmental, and individual factors as influences on healthy behavior.

- Behavioral (lifestyle) factors: Attitude, cultural values, religion, and a general level of education
- Environmental factors: Access to health services, socioeconomic conditions, quality of air, water, and soil
- Individual factors: Level of education, social status, and education on health issues

21

PRIMARY, SECONDARY, AND TERTIARY PREVENTION METHODS

Health educators distinguish between primary, secondary, and tertiary prevention methods:

- Primary prevention methods: Seek to avoid individual health problems
- Secondary prevention methods: Seek to diminish health problems in a population of individuals
- Tertiary prevention methods: Seek to mitigate the effects of a negative health condition on the individual level

CONDITIONS IMPACTING HEALTH EDUCATION

SOCIAL DETERMINANTS

Social determinants of health reflect social factors and the physical conditions in the environment in which people are born, live, learn, play, work, and age. Also known as social and physical determinants of health, they impact a wide range of health, functioning, and quality of life outcomes. Some illustrations of physical determinants include the following: natural environment (vegetation, climate), structures (buildings, means of transportation), workplaces, educational facilities, recreational facilities, neighborhoods (home structures/housing), physical hazards and toxins, barriers for those with disabilities, etc. Poor health outcomes may be made much worse by the interplay between individuals and the social/physical determinants of health.

SOCIAL CONDITIONS

Social conditions that may impact health education can be categorized as social institutions, surroundings, and social relationships. Social institutions can be cultural, religious, economic, and political. Surroundings can be the workplace, neighborhood, cities, and the "built environment." Social relationships can be social status or position, social groups, and networks. The Community Health Model recognizes that there are six social conditions that impact health outcomes. These social conditions are neighborhood conditions; learning opportunities; development of the community and available employment; current norms, customs, and established community processes; social cohesion; and health education and health promotion.

ENVIRONMENTAL CONDITIONS

As suggested by the ecological approach to health education/promotion, environmental conditions that may impact health education include the family, community, culture, physical environment, and social environment. The environmental factors that impact health education and health promotion are numerous and include an economy that enables choices that are health promoting, a society in which healthy choices and behaviors are recognized, educational information and the life skills to choose healthy behaviors and lifestyles, and an economy in which healthy goods and health services are readily available. Health education can have the best impact by allowing a population to exercise control over its environment.

FACTORS THAT ENHANCE OR COMPROMISE THE HEALTH EDUCATION PROCESS

Multiple factors can enhance or compromise the process of health education. It is important to determine the extent of available health education programs, interventions, and policies. One method to use to determine the extent of available programs, interventions, and policies is to conduct an administrative and policy assessment. Such an assessment yields information regarding the policies, available resources, and environment in an organized manner that will either enhance or compromise the development of a health education program. The administrative assessment serves to determine available personnel, available budget, and available time or time constraints.

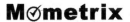

FACTORS PROMOTING OR DETRACTING FROM HEALTH EDUCATION

When health educators describe the factors that promote or detract from health education, they usually speak in terms of predisposing, enabling, and reinforcing factors. The ability to mitigate the impact of detracting factors while stimulating promoting factors is a product of knowledge and experience as a health educator.

- Predisposing factors: The assumptions and beliefs of the community concerning health issues
- Enabling factors: A willingness within the community to engage in positive health behavior changes
- Reinforcing factors: Presence of positive feedback for the purpose of solidifying positive changes in health behavior

FACTORS THAT FOSTER OR HINDER SKILL BUILDING

There are multiple factors that influence the learning process. Some factors that foster learning or skill building include the learning orientation of the participant and the individual's reason for participation. Learning orientation can be goal-oriented (education or skill used to attain a goal), activity-oriented (learn skill for the sake of the activity or social interaction), and learning-oriented (skill for the sake of knowledge). Factors that may hinder learning or skill building include external barriers and internal barriers. External barriers may be categorized as situational or institutional. Internal barriers may be categorized as dispositional.

An individual may participate in skill building to be social (meet new people), meet external demands (meet the demands of an authority), serve some social good (need to serve others or to serve the community as a whole), accomplish a professional achievement, for escape or stimulation (bored at work or at home), and to satisfy knowledge interest (learn for the sake of knowledge itself). Factors that might hinder learning or skill building include situational barriers (the individual's current situation), institutional barriers (policies, etc., of the institution), dispositional barriers (self-perception and perception regarding learning), geographic environment, age, gender (demographics), socioeconomic level, the level of education, and cultural expectations.

POLICY ASSESSMENT

Policy assessment is important when determining the extent of available policies in the process of health education. The policy assessment serves to ascertain the current policies or regulations and politics that may either enhance or may compromise the health education process and to promote existing policies, regulations, and programs that will facilitate the health education plan. A policy assessment requires that an assessment of the mission, etc., of the health education plan or process be compatible with existing regulations and policies and the amount of flexibility contained in such. It also serves to provide an assessment of the current political forces.

MEASURES TO ASSESS THE CAPACITY FOR IMPROVING COMMUNITY HEALTH STATUS

In order to set reasonable expectations for a health program, a health educator needs to honestly assess the capacity for improvement in community health status. This assessment will come in handy during the planning process, as health educators perform a needs assessment and resource inventory. Obviously, the amount of resources available for a program will directly contribute to its potential for improving health. Health educators may also want to look at the success records of similar, previous programs. Once a health educator has accurately assessed what needs to be done and what resources exist to do it, he or she can establish realistic expectations.

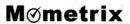

METHODS OF ASSESSMENT AND SYNTHESIZING FINDINGS

The behavioral and environmental assessment provides information regarding potential risk factors for the health problem, ranks the importance of the behavior, ranks change factors impacting the behavior, enables the selection of behaviors to target, and illustrates behavioral factors. The environmental assessment provides information as to the environmental risks contributing to the health problem, ranks the importance of the factors, changeability, identifies a target population, and illustrates the environmental factors. In order to synthesize the findings of the environmental assessment, the following criteria must be addressed: the correlation of the factor to the problem and the incidence, prevalence, or number of population affected.

IDENTIFICATION OF EMERGING HEALTH EDUCATION NEEDS

The educational and ecological assessment is highly useful in the identification of emerging health education needs. The educational and ecological assessment serves to identify causes linked to the health status or problem and to illustrate areas for change that require health education. The following factors are also identified and demonstrate areas for health educational needs: predisposing factors, enabling factors, and reinforcing factors. Predisposing factors are defined as antecedents to behavior that provide rationale or motivation for the behavior. Enabling factors are antecedents to behavior that allow the motivation to be realized. Reinforcing factors follow a behavior that provides continuing reward or incentive for the repetition of the behavior.

USING THE HEALTH GOALS SELECTED PHASE OF THE MATCH MODEL TO REPORT ASSESSMENT FINDINGS

The MATCH model is defined as "Multi-level Approaches to Community Health." The Health Goals Selected Phase of the MATCH model is one method in which to report assessment findings. The following steps are involved in the Health Goals Selected Phase: choose goals for health status and report the prevalence, change possibility, and resources available; choose the target population and report on the prevalence of the health issue in the target group, availability of the target population, and interest in the program; establish goals for health behavior; and establish goals for service access, program resources, and any restrictions.

GROUPING METHODS TERMS

- community forum: community members are assembled to discuss a particular health issue; these meetings are occasionally dominated by individuals with personal or specific issues, to the detriment of general discussion
- focus groups: specially-chosen individuals are assembled to discuss a particular issue; discussion is led by a facilitator; the results of a focus group must be considered in the light of the idiosyncratic composition of the group (i.e., focus groups typically do not represent the population as a whole)
- nominal group process: groups of five to seven people are assembled and asked to place the issues in question in a hierarchy, and then comment on those issues
- Delphi panels: members of the group complete three to five questionnaires, in increasing levels of specificity; health professionals read the responses and determine subsequent questions
- Self-assessment: individuals provide information about themselves; health professionals then compare this information with a known set of data

Plan Health Education/Promotion

PLANNING A HEALTH EDUCATION PROGRAM VS. THE PROGRAM ITSELF

When planning a health education program, a health professional will be assessing the needs and resources of the community in question. Planning must necessarily include an honest assessment of the limitations in a given situation, including any potential obstacles to the success of the program. The plan will need to include a list of all the health professionals that will be required for implementation of the program. Also, provisions should be made for training participants in the program and establishing a system of record keeping to document the success of the program. Once the health program is implemented, the focus of the planning health professional will be on evaluating its success. Success can only be defined as the extent to which the health education program meets the objectives for which it was originally created.

PLANNING AN EFFECTIVE HEALTH EDUCATION PROGRAM

Before an effective health education program can be implemented, it is important to accurately assess the health circumstances in the target community. The specific problems that need to be resolved must be clearly defined in order for the health education program to be on target. This may mean prioritizing the objectives of the health education program, so that secondary goals are not allowed to interfere with the primary goals. A clear eyed assessment should also include mention of any problems that are likely to endure the health education program. To complete an accurate assessment, health experts should be convened and relevant individuals in the community should be interviewed. Also, the planner should establish a clear system for record-keeping.

CHARACTERISTICS OF A PLAN FOR A HEALTH EDUCATION PROGRAM

In order to be considered professional, the plan for a health education program must be written down. It must include a summary of the program goals, all of the objectives that will contribute to the achievement of goals, and all of the particular tasks that will be required to meet each objective. It is essential that objectives be measurable so that the progress of the plan can be evaluated continuously. An effective and complete plan also needs to include a summary of the resources that will be required. Finally, the plan needs to include a summary of the data that will be used to measure the progress towards objectives.

IDENTIFYING STAKEHOLDERS IN THE ASSESSMENT PROCESS

A stakeholder may be defined as a person, group, or institution with interests in a project or policy or who may be directly or indirectly affected by the process or outcome. Identifying and analyzing stakeholders is an invaluable tool in gathering vital information as to which people will be impacted; which people may have influence or impact on the outcome; and which people, groups, or institutions need to be contacted for involvement. It helps identify the need to improve the participation of particular individuals, groups, or institutions. It is essential to ascertain key stakeholders early.

Stakeholder analysis is a vital tool to utilize when engaging stakeholders to participate in the assessment process. Such an analysis will provide critical information regarding the project environment and facilitate negotiation for discussion. Stakeholder analysis highlights the concerns and interests of various stakeholders regarding the areas to be addressed in the project in the planning phase, or in the objective of the project once it has begun. Analysis of stakeholders also helps to identify common ground between stakeholders, which may serve to further enhance the ability to proceed with the project.

25

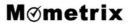

CREATING AN EFFECTIVE COALITION

Savvy health educators will constantly be forming coalitions within their target community. It is important, however, to make sure that these coalitions do not detract from the overall efforts of the health program. In other words, the terms of the coalition should not undermine the original intention of the health education program. One of the advantages of a coalition is that it has a broader base from which to draw manpower and financial assistance. Forming a coalition with a local civic organization, for instance, allows you to request financial assistance from all the members of that civic organization. Furthermore, individuals who have worked with that civic organization in the past will be more likely to contribute volunteer service or dollars to a program endorsed by the civic organization.

GETTING HELP AND SUPPORT WHEN PLANNING A HEALTH EDUCATION PROGRAM

In order to run a successful health education program, you'll need to receive support from organizations and individuals in the target community. Sometimes a health education program will require the financial resources of the business community; other times it might require the support of the education community. Sometimes there will be health experts in the area whose endorsements will be necessary to validate the intentions of the health education program. The best way to approach organizations and individuals whose help you need is to contact them in writing. Start off by declaring your intentions, and then describe the health issue and the purposes of your planned health program. In brief, summarize the ways in which the program will help to resolve the problem. Then, indicate how that individual or organization can contribute to the success of the program. Be sure to include your contact information.

COMMUNITY LEADERS HELPFUL IN IMPLEMENTING A HEALTH EDUCATION PROGRAM

It is always helpful to enlist the aid of community leaders when trying to spark the interest of the members of the target community. Health educators should send out query letters to any respected members of the community who might be able to positively influence their peers. Local charities, religious groups, and civic organizations are all potential sponsors of health education programs. One of the most important services that these partnerships can provide is publicity; being able to post information about your program at a local place of worship is a great way to get the word out. Also, working in collaboration with trusted and respected members of the community will validate your program in the eyes of the citizens. An endorsement from a community leader cannot be underestimated.

In order to be truly effective, a health education program needs to enlist the help of important and representative members of the target community. It is typical to first approach individuals and organizations in writing, clearly describing the intent of the health education program and the ways in which that individual or group could help. In the case of a tobacco education seminar, it would be important to contact local doctors, individuals who have suffered adverse health consequences of smoking, and any other relevant individuals. Be sure when writing to these individuals to include your name, organization, and contact information.

INVOLVING PEOPLE AND ORGANIZATIONS

A health education program vastly increases its potential for success when it actively involves people and organizations in the target community. In order to do this, a health instructor needs to know how to appeal to the self-interest of the individual or organization. When working with a business, for instance, a health educator needs to be able to demonstrate how improving health among employees will lead to greater productivity and fewer sick days. When working with individuals, a health instructor needs to be able to demonstrate how adherence to a behavior change will improve health and quality of life. The method of promotion will vary depending on the audience.

COMMUNITY-BASED ORGANIZATION

A community-based organization is defined as a public or private nonprofit organization of demonstrated effectiveness that is representative of a community or significant segments of a community, provides educational or related services to individuals in the community, can help solve a common problem or pursue a common goal, and helps community buy-in. By eliciting a community-based organization's support, opportunities for integrating health education are facilitated and supported. It is also important to use health communication in the community in conjunction with the community-based organization as a means of establishing support for further health education.

ELICITING INPUT FROM PRIORITY POPULATIONS

There are numerous methods by which to elicit input from priority populations and other stakeholders. Such methods include surveys, interviews, focus groups, direct observation, community forums, public meetings, nominal groups, Delphi panels, self-assessment instruments, a community capacity inventory, and community asset maps. The nominal group method is a data source using small groups of 5 to 7 people, each having an equal voice in the discussion and voting. All privately rank the ideas proposed and then share this ranking in a round-robin fashion. The Delphi panel utilizes questionnaires from decision makers, personnel, and participants in the program.

IMPORTANT COMPONENTS OF PROGRAM PLANNING

A health education program will never be successful unless it has a sound plan. In order to be comprehensive, a program plan needs to include a full list of goals and objectives, as well as the specific tasks that will enable these to be accomplished. These goals and objectives need to be realistic and in accord with the needs assessment. Also, it is essential to perform a comprehensive resource inventory before setting expectations for the program. The intervention method of the program should take into account the available resources, the prevailing attitudes among the target population, and the potential for assistance from other members of the community.

CONSIDERATIONS WHEN PROGRAM PLANNING

The health education program can only be effective if it is appropriate to the needs of the particular community. For instance, a smoking cessation program implemented in an area in which few residents smoke would be pointless. The health education program should be designed to resolve those problems in the community which are deemed to be the most egregious. Health education programs should be designed to make the maximum positive impact on the community. They should also include clear and measurable benchmarks that can be used to evaluate progress.

USING DATA AND ORGANIZATION TOGETHER TO SUCCEED

Although it is important to remain idealistic about the potential of health education programs, you will be better served if you base your decisions on the data and strong organization. Rather than trying to convert the target community to some ideal state, it is better to perform a thorough needs assessment and determine which specific, achievable goals can immediately improve health in some way. Unfortunately, health educators have to set priorities and focus on some problems to the exclusion of others. Also, they need to be realistic when setting expectations for their program; adequate attention to primary and secondary data during the needs assessment phase will enable health educators to establish reasonable expectations for their work.

MISSION STATEMENT

A mission statement is a brief explanation of the general intent of a health education program. It is composed so that members of the community can find out exactly why the health education program has been created. It is also supposed to help the members of the program stay on track and keep the original intentions in sight. Mission statements are usually only a sentence long, but in any case they are meant to be very short and memorable. A mission statement is often quite general, something along the lines of, "this health education program aims to improve the quality of life for the senior citizens in Montclair."

GOALS VS. OBJECTIVES IN PROGRAM PLANNING

When planning a health education program, it is important to establish *goals* and *objectives*. These are not the same thing. A goal is a general statement of long-term ambitions. For instance, the goal of the health education program might be to improve quality of life for senior citizens. Objectives, on the other hand, are specific achievements that must be attained in order to eventually meet the goals. Objectives have to be capable of measurement, and the system for measuring progress should be established during the planning phase. Objectives should include mention of who is responsible for each task, the length of time in which the task is to be completed, and the source of materials and resources for the completion of the task.

The *goals* of health education programs are general statements that indicate long term ambitions. In order to be effective, goals need to be clearly defined and measurable. Also, any stated goals should be in keeping with the mission statement of the program. Goals are often very general, as for instance, "this health program seeks to improve quality of life for the residents of the community." Other times, goals may be very specific, as for instance, "this health education program seeks to demonstrably reduce the adverse effects of smoking in the workplace." Goals may be financial, behavioral, or educational.

In a health education program, the *objectives* are those specific things that need to be accomplished in order to achieve a goal. Objectives have to be measurable and clearly defined. Also, explicit objectives must contain an explanation of who will be responsible for doing what, and in what timeframe. Objectives may be administrative, behavioral, learning, environmental, or program-oriented. For example, in order to reach a goal of improving fitness, one objective might be the ability to run a mile in less than 10 minutes.

PROGRAM OBJECTIVES

STATEMENT OF AN OBJECTIVE SHOULD INCLUDE AN ACTION VERB

When setting forth the objectives for a health education program, planners should take care to include an action verb so that the specific actions required to accomplish the objective will be known. Too often, objectives are set without any reference to the ways in which they will be accomplished. Including an action verb in the objective statement will also help to establish the appropriate indicator of progress. For instance, if the objective of a program fighting childhood obesity is to provide healthy food in schools, the administrative objective statement should explicitly state how that food is to be provided. The problem with imprecise words in an objective statement is that they leave too much room for interpretation, and do not establish a clear criterion for success.

EFFECTIVELY WRITTEN OBJECTIVES

In order to be effective, an objective must be explicit and clear. There should be a well defined system for evaluating the progress made towards achieving the objective. The system for

28

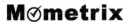

evaluating progress is known as an indicator. As a general rule, objectives should only have one indicator. Also, the amount of time in which the objective is to be completed should not be overly long. Objectives should always be the responsibility of participants in the health education program; in other words, planners should not set as an objective something over which they have no control. Finally, objectives need to be directly related to the overall goals of the program.

ADMINISTRATIVE OBJECTIVES

Health professionals establish administrative objectives to target their efforts for establishing a health education program. Specifically, administrative objectives are the organizational activities that will directly result in the success of the program. Sometimes, a health education program will include administrative objectives that define the set of rules and procedures that govern the behavior of the program. For example, an administrative objective might be to send out letters of inquiry to all local experts and important members of the community. Another administrative objective might be to establish a system for disseminating promotional literature.

IMPACT OBJECTIVES

Impact objectives are those things that must be done to lay the foundations for the achievement of the ultimate objectives of the health education program. Behavioral and learning objectives are the two most common kinds of impact objective. This is because changes must be made in behavior and knowledge before long term health goals can be achieved. In order to be effective, a written impact objective must include a description of the conditions in which it can be achieved, as well as the resources that will be required. An effective impact objective should also mention who will be responsible for achieving the objective. It is better to err on the side of making an objective too easy rather than too hard; unattainable objectives can be discouraging to participants.

BEHAVIORAL OBJECTIVES

Behavioral objectives are the changes in health-related behaviors that are the target of a health education program. For instance, one of the behavioral objectives of the day campaign against obesity would be increased frequency of cardiovascular exercise. It is important for behavioral objectives to be made explicit in the planning of the health education program, so that participants can take active steps to promote their achievement. Also, behavioral objectives have to be capable of being directly observed by health professionals. As much as possible, behavioral objectives should be measurable.

LEARNING OBJECTIVES

Learning (or instructional) objectives are changes in knowledge or skill that are the direct result of the successful implementation of a health education program. Programs that seek to promote awareness of a particular health issue will need to have learning objectives. Learning objectives are impact objectives, because they have a direct result on the quality of life of individuals. It is especially important when writing a learning objective to make sure that it is clear and explicit; an increase in knowledge may be subtle, so there must be appropriate indicators of progress. Most research suggests that in order to sustain positive changes in health behavior, individuals must obtain some amount of knowledge on the subject in question.

PROGRAM OBJECTIVES

Health professionals set program objectives (also known as outcome objectives) that define exactly what service is to be provided to the community in question. A well-written program objective will also indicate the timeframe in which this service is to be delivered. For example, a program to fight childhood obesity might declare that it will provide healthy alternatives to junk food in schools

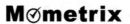

within the next year. Program objectives should specifically mention the actions that will directly result in success, and should include a clearly-defined indicator for measuring progress.

ENVIRONMENTAL OBJECTIVES

An environmental objective is some change in the physical or social environment that will positively affect health. For example, a health education program concerned with promoting fitness might have as an environmental objective more playground equipment for small children. The presence of more playground equipment would promote exercise. This is an environmental objective that seeks to influence individual behavior; other environmental objectives will not have anything to do with behavior. For instance, a program that aims to reduce asbestos might set as an objective the removal of certain kinds of insulation within one year.

SCENARIO ONE

You are a health educator for International Conglomerate. The mission of the company's health program is to foster a workforce that is healthy in body, mind, and spirit.

1. Explain why the following is not an appropriate goal, and then take steps to make it suitable for inclusion in the program:

   Company employees will stay healthy.

   The statement "company employees will stay healthy" is not appropriate as a goal for health education because it is too vague. Even though goals are broad statements indicating the long-term intentions of a program, they still need to be phrased with enough precision that they can be evaluated. Specifically, the definition of "healthy" is too nebulous to serve as a true target. The health education program needs to establish a specific definition of health before setting it as a goal. So, an improved statement will be one that succinctly but precisely establishes the criterion for success. For instance, the example statement might be improved by changing it to "Company employees will spend less time in the infirmary."

2. Explain why the following is not an appropriate program objective, and then take steps to make it suitable for inclusion in the program:

   International Conglomerate will make sure employees understand the dangers of smoking.

   Program objectives, a kind of health objective, are statements defining the precise services that are to be provided to the target community. In order to be complete, a program objective also needs to include the timeframe in which the objective is to be achieved. The program objective should indicate the way in which progress will be measured. The program objective, "International Conglomerate will make sure employees understand the dangers of smoking" fails because it does not include a standard for evaluation. There is no time frame, and the definition of employee understanding is not specified. A better program objective statement would be the following: "International Conglomerate will increase employee exposure to anti-smoking literature over the next year."

3. Explain why the following is not an appropriate outcome objective, and then take steps to make it suitable for inclusion in the program:

    Smoking-related illnesses among employees of International Conglomerate will decrease.

Outcome objectives are another form of health objectives. An outcome objective statement defines the change in health quality that will be accomplished by the success of a health education program. As with other objective statements, an outcome objective is not complete unless it contains a timeframe and a clear system of evaluation. The outcome objective statement should contain an action verb that specifically indicates what must be done for the objective to be accomplished. The outcome objective statement, "Smoking-related illnesses among employees of International Conglomerate will decrease" does not include a timeframe. Also, the statement could be improved by indicating the exact target amount of the decrease. For instance, the statement could be rewritten as follows: "Smoking-related illness among employees of International Conglomerate will decrease by 20% over the next five years."

4. Explain why the following is not an appropriate behavioral objective, and then take steps to make it suitable for inclusion in the program:

    International Conglomerate employees who complete a smoking cessation program will understand how to remain smoke-free.

Behavioral objectives are a form of impact objective. They outline the changes in behavior in the target community that will lead to the accomplishments of health-related goals. In order to be complete, the statement of their behavioral objective needs to include the conditions under which the change in behavior will be accomplished and the precise level of change required. It is not necessary for a behavioral objective statement to include a timeframe. The behavioral objective statement "International Conglomerate employees who complete a smoking cessation program will understand how to remain smoke-free" does not imply a system for evaluation. Also, it offers no way to define employee understanding. A better way to rewrite this statement would be as follows: "International Conglomerate employees will utilize strategies to avoid smoking after they have participated in a smoking-cessation program."

5. Explain why the following is not an appropriate administrative objective, and then take steps to make it suitable for inclusion in the program:

    Assess the contents of each vending machine on an hourly basis to make sure nicotine gum is available.

An administrative objective is an outline of the tasks and plans that need to be accomplished in order to meet the larger objectives and goals of the health education program. In order to be successful, a health education program must be effectively organized. The statement of an administrative objective should include an action verb indicating what needs to be done as well as how progress will be measured. Also, administrative objectives must be within the realm of possibility.

For instance, the statement "Assess the contents of each vending machine on an hourly basis to make sure nicotine gum is available" places an unreasonable demand on participants. It is unlikely that gum will be sold fast enough for hourly checks to be necessary. A more appropriate administrative objective would be "Check the vending machines every day to make sure nicotine gum is available."

6. Explain why the following is not an appropriate learning objective, and then take steps to make it suitable for inclusion in the program:

   International Conglomerate employees will be aware of how smoke moves through the body from inhalation to exhalation.

   Instructional objectives are a form of impact objective. An instructional objective outlines the specific changes in understanding and skill that will enable behavioral objectives to be accomplished. Research indicates time and again that permanent behavioral changes are much more likely when the individual has a knowledge base upon which to rely. As for all other statements of objective, the statement of an instructional objective must include an action verb, a reasonable desired outcome, and a clear method of evaluation. The statement "International Conglomerate employees will be aware of how smoke moves through the body from inhalation to exhalation" fails to meet these criteria. There is no precise definition of awareness, so it will be impossible to measure the progress towards meeting the subjective. A more effective instructional objective statement could be the following: "After completing a smoking cessation program, International Conglomerate employees will be able to pass a short exam on the path of smoke through the human body from inhalation to exhalation."

DECIDING WHAT INFORMATION SHOULD BE INCLUDED IN AN EDUCATION PROGRAM

In order to be effective, an education program needs to contain all of the necessary information but none of the superfluous or irrelevant information. When commentators refer to a health educator as a clearinghouse, they are referring to the responsibility of a health educator to survey all the available information on the subject and choose for dissemination only the most essential. For instance, the educator will want to abstain from distributing any promotional literature that is either too sophisticated or too simplistic for the target audience. The educator will also have to keep in mind the budget limitations that may constrain the amount of information that can be distributed.

SCENARIO TWO

You have been hired to develop a health education program for students, faculty and staff at State University.

1. Outline the general process you would use.

   Before implementation of a health education program can begin, it's important to assess the overall health status of the target community and determine what sort of health education program would be most beneficial. To this end, health professionals should assemble data and interview members of the community before planning begins. After the general focus of the health education program has been established, specific goals should be decided upon. Then, health professionals should determine which specific objectives must be accomplished in order to reach those long-term goals. All of the activities of the health education program should be directly related to the achievement of these objectives. Also, a resource inventory needs to be performed.

2. Keeping in mind that any program should be geared toward changing specific behaviors to improve the health of a community, give appropriate examples of the following elements: mission statement, goal, program objective, outcome objective, impact objective (behavioral), impact objective (learning), administrative objective.

   Additional elements:

   - Mission statement: The student health center at State University seeks to improve quality of life for all members of the community.
   - Goal: The student health center will work with students on an individual and group basis to improve health.
   - Program objective: State University will establish a smoking-cessation program on campus.
   - Outcome objective: Tobacco use among State University students will decrease by 10% within the next three years.
   - Impact objective (behavioral): All incoming students will be required to attend a seminar on tobacco use.
   - Impact objective (learning): Students who attend the seminar must be able to identify the health risks associated with smoking.
   - Administrative objective: The student health center will host guest speakers from the medical community.

MATCH MODEL VS. PRECEDE-PROCEED MODEL

Health educators typically use either the MATCH or the PRECEDE-PROCEED model when planning a program. The MATCH model consists of five phases, with an emphasis on selecting the appropriate kind of intervention for a particular community. This model is especially popular when implementing the program for a large group of people. The PRECEDE-PROCEED model, on the other hand, consists of nine phases running from needs assessment and diagnosis to implementation and evaluation. This method is generally used when implementing a long-term program for a specific population. It focuses on establishing an environment conducive to permanent positive behavior change.

The PRECEDE-PROCEED model of health education program planning is composed of nine phases for diagnosis, implementation, and evaluation. To begin with, planners perform a social diagnosis, in which information about the target community is gathered and analyzed. At this point, there are no strictly defined goals and objectives for the health education program. As information is gathered and organized, planners will decide which specific health problems need to be addressed, and how this can be best accomplished. The MATCH system for health education planning, meanwhile, moves from diagnosis to implementation in only five phases. This system is appropriate for health education programs that will require an intervention.

PRECEDE-PROCEED, MATCH:

- PRECEDE-PROCEED: stands for Predisposing, Reinforcing, Enabling Constructs in Educational/Ecological Diagnosis and Evaluation—Policy, Regulatory, and Organizational Constructs in Educational and Environmental Development; In this system, needs are identified, plans are constructed (PRECEDE), programs are activated, and evaluations are made (PROCEED); PRECEDE has four phases, PROCEED has five phases

- MATCH: stands for Multilevel Approach To Community Health; Consists of five phases, beginning with the identification of goals and ending with assessing the success of the program; typically used when the health education program requires a direct intervention

PHASES OF THE PRECEDE PORTION OF THE PRECEDE-PROCEED MODEL

- Phase 1: Social assessment: A collection of pertinent information is assembled; should include all salient facts about the health issue in question
- Phase 2: Epidemiological assessment: Assembled data is scrutinized for patterns and trends; experts determine the correlation between health problems and the environment in which the community lives
- Phase 3: Behavioral assessment: List is made of activities and environmental factors that contribute to the health issue
- Phase 4: Educational and ecological assessment: Health professionals determine the extent to which educational factors, like health awareness and promotion, contribute to the health issue

PHASES OF THE PROCEED PORTION OF THE PRECEDE-PROCEED MODEL

- Phase 5: Administrative and policy assessment: Health professionals calculate the resources that are required and available for implementation of the health education program
- Phase 6: Implementation: Results of the assessments performed in the PRECEDE process are put into action; a comprehensive health education program includes attention to the social and behavioral influences on health
- Phase 7: Process evaluation: A comprehensive health education program includes a system for evaluating the success of each component after implementation
- Phase 8: Impact evaluation: Assessment of the extent to which the program is educating the public, as well as a summary of any general changes in the health-related behavior of the community
- Phase 9: Outcome evaluation: Overall evaluation of the extent to which the health education program achieved its original goals

PHASES OF THE MATCH (MULTILEVEL APPROACH TO COMMUNITY HEALTH) MODEL

MATCH is a comprehensive system for the planning, implementation, and evaluation of a health education program. It includes five distinct phases.

- Phase 1: Goal selection: Long-term health goal and secondary behavioral and environmental goals are defined
- Phase 2: Intervention planning: Target and objectives of intervention are established; intervention approach is selected based on the circumstances in which it will be performed
- Phase 3: Program development: Elements of the health education program are produced; these may include promotional literature, visual aids for presentations, and training manuals for staff
- Phase 4: Implementation preparation: Participants in the health education program are selected and trained, program is put into action
- Phase 5: Evaluation: According to a previously-established system, the program is evaluated and corrected as necessary

SCENARIO THREE

Several State University students have recently been arrested for DUI. The University has now asked you to plan a health education program that will reduce, if not eliminate, the problem.

Explain why you will use the planning process laid out by MATCH (Multilevel Approach To Community Health) rather than the one involved in PRECEDE-PROCEED.

Health professionals typically use the MATCH planning process when an intervention is necessary. In this case, it is clear that the serious nature of the problem calls for a direct intervention. Specifically, the University has declared that drunk driving arrests must be severely diminished if not entirely eliminated. For this reason, the MATCH system would be more appropriate. One advantage of this system is that it contains fewer phases and can be executed more quickly. The five phases of the MATCH system are as follows: goal selection, intervention planning, program development, implementation preparation, and evaluation. The other system for planning a health education program, known as the PRECEDE-PROCEED system, is more effective for identifying the distinct factors that can contribute to a complex health problem.

CDCYNERGY MODEL

CDCynergy is a tool for developing health communications and interventions. It was developed by the Centers for Disease Control and Prevention. It is based on a CD-ROM platform. The program operates by asking the user a series of questions designed to isolate the message to be publicized or the tasks to be accomplished. It aims to streamline the process of program organization by offering a ready-made template for data and ideas. The CDCynergy model contains planning, implementation, and evaluation assistance. This model is especially effective at generating a clear program plan in a short amount of time.

LOGICAL MODEL

A logical model is defined as a logical series of statements that link problems the program is attempting to address (conditions), how it will address them (activities), and the expected results (immediate, intermediate, and long-term goals). A logical model functions as a guide to planning a program. A logic model may also gauge the efficiency and efficacy of the program because it contains the following measures: inputs, outputs, actions, outcomes, and the program impact. Other models that may be used include: MATCH model and CDCynergy.

SOCIAL COGNITIVE THEORY

The social cognitive theory promotes the concept that learning is an interplay between the person, environment, and cognitive and behavioral factors. The social cognitive theory integrates, therefore, approaches to behavioral change by using cognitive, behavioral, and environmental aspects. The following are the nine constructs of the social cognitive theory: reciprocal determinism, self-efficacy, behavioral capability, outcome expectation, outcome expectancies, performance self-control, observational learning, environment and situations, and reinforcement. Reciprocal determinism is how the person, environment, and behavior interact and influence each other. Self-efficacy is the confidence one has in performing a behavior.

TRANSTHEORETICAL MODEL OF CHANGE (TTM)

The transtheoretical model of change (TTM) utilizes interventions that are designed to impact individuals at the stage in which they are regarding change. The TTM uses the aspects of many different health education theories. The TTM has four constructs: stages of change, decisional balance, self-efficacy, and change processes. The stages of change in the TTM are as follows: precontemplation (not planning to change at all in next 6 months), contemplation (planning to change in next 6 months), preparation (plan to take action in next 30 days), action (behavior change for 6 months), maintenance (behavior change for over 6 months with efforts to prevent relapse), and termination (no risk of relapse).

ENSURING THAT HEALTH COMMUNICATION STRATEGIES WILL BEST MEET PROGRAM OBJECTIVES

In order for health communication strategies to meet program objectives, they must be appropriate to both the target population and to the goals and objectives of the program. The medium of communication needs to be one that is appropriate to the population; for instance, it would not make sense to place health communications for junior high school students in the daily newspaper. Similarly, a health communication must be specifically designed to meet the goals and objectives of the particular health education program. For instance, a smoking cessation program should concentrate its message on the dangers of smoking, rather than encouraging exercise as an indirect way of decreasing tobacco use.

Strategies available for meeting objectives of a health education program:

- Health related community service strategies: Free or low-cost services or screenings
- Health communication strategies: promotion and dissemination of health issues through the media
- Community mobilization: Efforts to involve the target community through advocacy and the building of coalitions
- Health engineering strategies: Efforts to positively alter the elements of the physical environment that affect health
- Educational strategies: Efforts to inform the target population about a specific health issue
- Health policy or enforcement strategies: efforts to influence behavior through changes in government or organizational policy

SELECTING APPROPRIATE REFERENCES

One of the problems that health educators currently face is an overabundance of health references. It is increasingly important to be able to cull the most important statistics and reference information for the development of a health education program. Health educators need to be familiar with the statistical reports put out by the US Census Bureau, the National Center for Health Statistics, and the Office of Disease Prevention and Health Promotion. All of these organizations provide a service to health educators by assembling only the most important data and research results for the development of health education programs.

FACILITATING AND PROMOTING THE LEARNING PROCESS

At all times, health educators should be searching for ways to make the learning process easier for the members of the target audience. The best and most obvious way to do this is to stay abreast of the progress being made through constant assessment. This assessment may take the form of formal examinations, but it can also be accomplished through informal conversations and surveys. As much as possible, health educators should make the location welcoming and encouraging to students. Also, health educators should use a variety of instructional strategies to account for students with different learning styles.

The most important thing you can do to improve learning among the target population is to increase motivation. Of course, this is easier said than done. There are a few ways, however, to promote learning. One way is to encourage individuals to become active participants in the education process. Group discussions and collaborative meetings are better at engaging reluctant students than are lectures. Although it is important to provide adequate promotional literature, it is also important to give individuals visual instruction as well. You cannot rely on uninterested students to closely read health education literature. In some cases, videos and slide presentations can be an effective way to disseminate important information.

TARGET POPULATION NOT INTERESTED IN LEARNING

When dealing with a population that is unwilling to learn essential health information, a health professional has to rely on all sorts of tricks of the trade. Some health educators try to help people learn by engaging them in a hypothetical situation or role-play; others make a game out of learning in the hopes of inspiring their students. As much as possible, the members of the target population should be encouraged to become personally involved in the learning process; research consistently suggests that individuals learn better when they feel they have a stake in the subject. A health educator should constantly evaluate the success of his or her methods, making adjustments when necessary.

Principles that can be used to promote the learning process:

- Increase or decrease the speed of presentation depending on the difficulty of the material
- Encourage students to apply class material to their own lives
- Begin with known premises and work to unknown conclusions
- Maintain a positive learning environment
- Present difficult information in a variety of ways
- Demonstrate the connections between seemingly disparate topics
- Make sure students are comfortable
- Engage students in regular class discussions

TARGET POPULATION INABILITY TO UNDERSTAND

Sometimes, health education will require you to teach detailed and complex information to the target population. In order to simplify a complicated subject as much as possible, break it down into its constituent elements and teach these individually. Make sure that all of your students have the necessary educational background to understand the material; it is important not to alienate students by talking over their heads. For especially complex subjects, you may want to present the same information in a variety of different ways, for instance visually, through class discussion, and through a text. As much as possible, students should be encouraged to become active participants in the educational process.

TAILORED MESSAGE

When health educators refer to a "tailored message," they are referring to a message that has been specifically adapted for the target population. A comprehensive needs assessment is the foundation of an appropriate tailored message, but health educators also need to determine the medium of presentation that will be most effective in reaching the target audience. Also, health educators will have to select the practical information that is most appropriate for the target audience; encouraging senior citizens to initiate vigorous exercise, for instance, is a less effective way of improving health and encouraging subtle changes in diet.

LEARNING ACTIVITIES

When health educators use the phrase "learning activities," they are referring to those actions which intend to improve knowledge and skills in the target community. All of the learning activities in a health education program should be designed for the accomplishment of the learning objectives. Learning activities can be as simple as handing out health-related literature, or as involved as leading a community meeting. Learning activities are only successful if the target population can be encouraged to engage with them.

HEALTH EDUCATION PLANNING FOR DIFFERENT AUDIENCES

In order to be effective as a health educator, you will need to tailor your message for different audiences. When working in a community, for instance, you'll need to actively engage the target population. In a health care facility, on the other hand, you can assume that the individuals with whom you will be dealing will already have a certain amount of interest in your program. When planning programs in colleges and universities, you should be focusing on preventive care and education, as students will be more inclined to take an active role in the maintenance of good health. One rapidly expanding field for health education is business, where the employer is likely to ask you to target a specific portion of the population for a specific purpose.

ACHIEVING STATED OBJECTIVES

It is vital to use the strategy of organization at the grassroots level to engage the target population as well as stakeholders. Community organization is essentially a six-step process: recognizing the problem in the community, utilizing health education specialists to organize the target population and stakeholders, assessing the community, establishing priorities, choosing interventions and means of implementation, and analyzing and continually assessing the formulated plan of action. Another effective strategy is to form a coalition. There are seven steps in forming a coalition: analyzing the problem, generating awareness, establishing planning and recruitment for the coalition, obtaining funding and other resources, establishing infrastructure and leadership, and generating an action plan.

ETHICAL PRINCIPLES AND LEGAL STANDARDS TO CONSIDER WHEN PLANNING AN INTERVENTION

ANA's Code of Ethics and the AHA's Patient's Bill of Rights guide **ethical practice** for interventions in health education. Ethical principles include respect for autonomy, the person's right to self-determination. This principle is supported by the Patient Self-Determination Act (1992), which requires all healthcare facilities to comply with this act's regulations. Veracity, truth telling, is part of informed consent and is essential to health education. Informed consent requires that the person be competent to give consent; has been apprised of risks, benefits, and alternatives; comprehends the information provided; and gives consent without coercion. The principle of confidentiality is supported by the Health Information Portability and Accountability Act (HIPAA), which requires that all personal information about a patient must be kept private and secure. The health education specialist should intervene under the principles of nonmalfeasance (doing no harm) as failure to uphold this principle can lead to legal actions for negligence or malpractice. The health education specialist should practice under the principles of beneficence (doing good) and justice (fairness and equal distribution).

DEVELOPING AND MONITORING A TIMELINE

Developing a **timeline** requires making a list of all tasks and the steps involved and then placing the tasks in sequential order. For each task, the necessary resources and the time needed to carry out the task should be estimated. A timeline can be developed manually, but it this can be very time-consuming, especially because modifications are frequently needed. For his reason, software applications are often used in development of timelines. Gantt charts provide visual representations of tasks and the time needed for each tasks as well as overlapping tasks. Other methods used include the critical path method, which is a network diagramming technique that helps to determine time needed and the earliest completion time; critical chain scheduling, which identifies constraints and builds in time buffers; and Program Evaluation and Review Technique (PERT), which is a valuable time estimation tool when time needed for individual tasks is uncertain. The timeline should be continuously monitored throughout the planning and implementation phases and adjusted as necessary.

SOCIAL MARKETING AND HEALTH COMMUNICATION ROLES

Social marketing is simply the application of commercial marketing principles to a health related problem. The practice of social marketing emerged in the 1970s when health educators realized that they could incorporate the insights of marketing to further their own work. Basically, social marketing is the process of persuading a target audience to adopt changes in their health behavior. Health communication is a similar effort, in which educators try to disseminate health information through the media. The intention of both social marketing and health communication efforts is to engage citizens in health-related issues by showing them how these issues directly affect their lives.

INTEGRATING HEALTH EDUCATION INTO OTHER PROGRAMS

There are predisposing factors and reinforcing factors to be used in the process of integrating health education into other programs. Predisposing factors or resources to be considered include using mass media (surveys, focus groups), local media sources, organization sponsors (political, governmental, corporate), and interpersonal communication implemented by training and educating personnel. Reinforcing factors or resources to be considered include garnering organizational support via continuous staff training and education; developing leadership via teacher training, parent education, and training of community leaders; and instituting peer groups to facilitate continued health education.

ASSESSMENT OF THE SUSTAINABILITY OF A HEALTH EDUCATION PLAN OR PROMOTION

Sustainability should be an issue dealt with in all phases of planning for a health education plan or promotion. Issues to consider related to sustainability include:

- Need: The need for the plan is the primary consideration. Some education plans/promotions are time-limited and may not be ongoing, but it's more cost-effective if plans can be sustained with modifications as needed over longer periods of time because planning and implementation can be time-consuming or costly.
- Resources: A plan or promotion cannot be sustained if the financial support and resources (materials, equipment, staff, space) are not available, so this must be a consideration when prioritizing issues in the initial planning stages.
- Support: Administrative and Board support for a plan is often critical because these individuals allocate resources.
- Currency: Education plans or promotions with built-in obsolescence (such as a program focusing out outgoing technology or healthcare practice) are not sustainable.

FACTORS AFFECTING THE IMPLEMENTATION OF A HEALTH EDUCATION PLAN

The two main factors that affect the implementation of a health education plan are available resources and potential barriers. A health education program can only be effective to the extent that it has the resources it needs. Health plans that set unreasonably high expectations are just as counterproductive as those that set the bar too low. Money and manpower are the two most

39

important resources for health education program; without sufficient amounts of each, the program will never live up to its plans. As for potential barriers, these may include the aforementioned lack of resources, conflict between staff members, and a lack of communication and corporation with members of the community. These barriers should be acknowledged and strategies should be devised for overcoming them as soon as possible.

TYPES OF RESULT AND EVALUATION OBJECTIVES

- administrative objectives: organized, streamlined administrative processes for administering services; evaluated by determining the contributions of staff, and the appropriateness of administrative procedures for the particular task
- learning objectives: changes in knowledge or skills on the part of the target population; evaluated through quizzes, interviews, and indirect observation
- behavioral objectives: observable changes in health behavior on the part of the target population; evaluated through interviews and observation
- environmental objectives: changes in the elements of the environment that affect health; evaluated by observation and direct measurement
- program objectives: changes in health and quality of life among the target population; evaluated by determining the degree to which the overall objectives of the program are being met

PLANNING HEALTH EDUCATION PROGRAM TERMS

- stakeholders: all those individuals who will be influenced by a health education program
- social marketing: the means of publicizing and promoting a health education program to the members of the target community
- health communication: the general practice of disseminating health information to the target population, with the hope of making positive changes in the lives of stakeholders
- programs: the organized distribution of health-related services to a specific population
- program planning: the process of designing the organization, implementation, and evaluation of a health education program; must be comprehensive and highly detailed if the program is to succeed
- community-based organization (CBO): a non-profit organization designed to improve life for the members of a community by providing some service, like healthcare, education, or
- mission statement: succinct summary of the program; includes a description of the purpose
- goal: a broad statement of the long term ambitions of the health education program
- objective: the specific achievements that will contribute to the realization of the goal; in order to be professional, an objective must include a system for measuring its own achievement; activities, resources, and planning efforts are designed to meet the objectives

Implement Health Education/Promotion

IMPLEMENTATION

When health educators use the term "implementation," they are referring to the process of putting health education program plans into action. The implementation of a program is the initiation of those activities which intends to bring about a specific change in health and the target population. Implementation includes the establishment of a system for evaluating the progress of the program. Effective implementation requires the participation of the target population, as well as the requisite resources and man power.

The first phase of any program implementation is to somehow encourage the target population to take an interest in the program. Without some degree of community interest, the health education program has no chance of success. So, health educators need to take specific steps to draw members of the community into the program. Perhaps the best way to do this is to demonstrate the importance of the health issue to the personal life of each member of the community. When the members of the target community feel that they have a personal stake in the success of the health program, they are more likely to contribute to its success.

After health professionals have taken steps to develop community interest in the education program, they will move on to the second phase of the implementation process: conducting a resource and task inventory. Many health professionals make use of the established planning methods PERT (Program Evaluation and Review Technique) or MBO (Management By Objectives) during this phase. In any case, it is necessary to compile a complete list of all the materials and activities that will be required for the accomplishment of the program goals. Resources may include money, people, and equipment.

After the completion of a resource and task inventory, health professionals can move on to the third phase of the implementation process: program planning. During this phase, health professionals will determine the precise set and sequence of activities that will result in the success of the program. This is done by defining the objectives that must be reached in order to meet program goals and then by listing those activities that will enable the accomplishment of the program objectives. It is essential that the program plan include a timetable and a system for evaluation. Responsibility should be clearly delegated, and the sources of money and equipment should be predetermined.

After completing an extensive program plan, health educators can move on to the fourth phase of the implementation process: putting those plans into action. This can be done in a variety of ways. In some cases, as with new and untested programs, it is best to put part of the plan into action and conduct an evaluation. This is known as a trial run or pilot study. Other plans, however, can be implemented all at once. Obviously, the faster a program can be implemented in its entirety, the faster it will be able to deliver all the intended services.

Even after program plans have been implemented, the work of health educators is not complete; it is still necessary to maintain a constant evaluation of the program and to make helpful adjustments. The fifth and final phase of the implementation process is using this evaluation to decide whether to terminate the program or continue it. Programs must be allowed to operate for a reasonable amount of time before they are judged to be insufficient. However, programs that show no sign of meeting their goals should not be continued in perpetuity. It is a good idea to establish a trial period for the program at its inception.

41

COORDINATION TASKS

There are a few different tasks that a health educator must perform in order to effectively coordinate the implementation of a health education program. To begin with, the health educator needs to organize and administrate effective training programs for all members of staff. The health educator also needs to establish a system for communication among various parties. Holding regular meetings is one way to encourage a continuous flow of information through the members of the program. Similarly, the health educator needs to make sure that relationships between various participants in the program are professional and productive. Finally, the health educator needs to ensure that all necessary resources are available to staff.

ISSUES WHEN CHOOSING METHODS

At all times, health educators should take care to make sure that the activities in a health education program are safe, legal, and ethical. Equipment and facilities used for the programs should be examined to ensure their safety, and students should never be required to participate in activities that they fear may threaten their health. There should always be access to medical personnel and first-aid equipment. As for legal concerns, the participants in a health education program should sign an informed consent waiver before beginning the program. This document will outline the activities and issues that will be covered during the program. Finally, health educators need to abide by their Code of Ethics and avoid any behaviors that diminish their ability to promote health education.

EDUCATIONAL ACTIVITIES USED TO IMPLEMENT A HEALTH EDUCATION PROGRAM

There are a variety of educational activities that can be incorporated into a health education program. For instance, many health educators use visual presentations like films or slideshows to draw interest. For some subjects, there is no substitute for a textbook or pamphlet. In some cases, it may be appropriate to lead a field trip. For instance, a health education program aimed at increasing awareness of nutrition might benefit from a field trip to the local farmers' market. In order to keep students engaged in the educational process, teachers may want to include workshops and seminars as part of the education program.

INFLUENCE OF DIFFERENT ENVIRONMENTS ON THE ADMINISTRATION OF HEALTH EDUCATION PROGRAMS

As a health educator, you will need to learn how to function effectively in different work environments. If you are working in a school, you will have to coordinate your efforts with the school administration. You will also have to abide by the rules and restrictions of the school system. If you are working in a private health care facility, on the other hand, you will have to coordinate your efforts with the work of doctors and nurses. If you are working in a community, you will have to work harder to engage the interest of the target population, who will not be required or feel they have any incentive to help you.

COORDINATING AN INTERVENTION ROLES

Oftentimes, a health intervention will require the close coordination of a number of independent parts. With knowledge and experience, a health educator can make the implementation of a program as smooth as possible. In order to do this, however, the health educator needs to make sure that communication between team members is easy and frequent. The health educator also needs to make sure that sufficient resources are available, and that all participants are fully trained and understand their jobs.

USING THE CODE OF ETHICS IN PROFESSIONAL PRACTICE

Obviously, health educators need to keep the code of ethics in mind in all aspects of their professional practice. Some health issues, particularly those related to birth control and sexually transmitted diseases, are especially controversial and need to be handled with discretion. Another important ethical concern is informed consent and privacy considerations. The code of ethics provides a specific set of guidelines for handling these and other potential ethical pitfalls in the profession.

The Code of Ethics for the Health Education Profession has six articles, outlining the general responsibilities of a health educator. They are as follows:

1. Responsibility to the public
2. Responsibility to the profession
3. Responsibility to employers
4. Responsibility in the delivery of health education
5. Responsibility in research evaluation
6. Responsibility in professional preparation

ARTICLE I

Article I of the code of ethics deals with the responsibility that a health educator has to the public. Specifically, health educators are meant to teach people ways to improve their own health and the health of members of their community. It is especially important, however, to give adequate autonomy to each individual; in other words, health educators are not to use coercive methods to force individuals to change their behavior. As much as possible, individuals should be encouraged to change their own behavior voluntarily. Health educators are required to provide services without discrimination and to respect the privacy of those individuals with whom they work.

ARTICLE II

The second article of the code of ethics deals with a health educator's responsibility to the profession. In order for health educators to maintain their good reputation in the community, they need to abide by a strict moral code. Health educators need to also monitor the behavior of their peers and intervene when they believe the highest standards of the profession are being violated. One way for health educators to promote their profession is by joining a professional organization. Another is to publicize their own work and the work of others.

ARTICLE III

The third article of the code of ethics deals with the responsibility that a health educator has to his or her employer. Health educators need to respect the desires of their bosses and strive to do their very best to serve the interest of the organization with which they are affiliated. In order to do this, health educators need to be very clear with their employers about any possible conflicts of interest. They also need to give honest evaluations of their work, so that their employers can make good decisions. Sometimes, it is necessary for a health educator to honestly admit that a program is not succeeding.

ARTICLE IV

The fourth article of the code of ethics describes the responsibility of a health educator to deliver instruction in an effective and appropriate manner. Health educators have to work with all kinds of people, so they need to have a full repertoire of instructional strategies and materials to make their work effective in different contexts. This means keeping in mind any legal issues, especially those

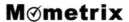

related to diversity. Health educators must furnish informed consent forms whenever appropriate, so that participants in a health program will be aware of the benefits and risks.

ARTICLE V

The fifth article of the code of ethics describes the responsibility of a health educator to perform research and evaluation ethically. There are typically laws, professional standards, and local regulations that constrain research methods. Health educators need to make sure that all participants in a health program are there voluntarily and have filled out any relevant informed consent documents. Health educators should make sure the credit for research and evaluation is given to the appropriate party, and that evaluation is as accurate and unbiased as possible.

ARTICLE VI

The sixth article of the code of ethics describes the responsibility of a health educator to be fully prepared to discharge his or her professional duties. Health educators need to treat their students with respect and to seek out those instructional methods that can best deliver important information. The learning environment needs to be inclusive and welcoming for all students. Course material needs to be current and accurate. Any evaluations made of students need to be fair and objective.

> **Review Video: Organizational Ethics**
> Visit mometrix.com/academy and enter code: 885880

REDUCING THE LIKELIHOOD OF LEGAL PROBLEMS

The best way to avoid legal problems as a health educator is to be knowledgeable on potential issues and abreast of related legislation. Health educators need to be conscious of when they are liable or responsible for a student's safety. All participants in a health education program should be given an informed consent document at the program's initiation. This document should detail the activities that will make up the program, including any potential risks. Health educators should only perform those activities for which they have been trained.

There are a few legal issues that must be considered when planning and implementing a health education program. For one thing, participants should sign an informed consent waiver indicating that they understand the content and intention of the program. The informed consent waiver should include any and all information pertaining to the activities and materials to be used in the program. Any risks associated with the program should be declared in the informed consent waiver. The participants in a health education program are dependent on the health professional in charge, and in turn, he or she is responsible for them. Health educators are subject to charges of negligence if they fail to perform their duties adequately.

ETHICAL ISSUES

There are a number of ethical considerations common to the life of a health educator. Indeed, a health educator needs to pay attention to professional ethics throughout the planning and implementation of a program. According to the professional code of ethics, the basic principles of responsible health education are respecting the autonomy of the individual, promoting health and wellness, avoiding activities that could potentially harm the target community, and promoting social justice in general.

SAFETY ISSUES

A health educator needs to pay special attention to safety concerns when implementing a health education program. All appropriate caution should be taken to minimize risk for participants. To

44

begin with, health professionals should survey the setting of the program and assess its safety. The area needs to be well lit, in a safe area of town, and needs to have adequate access to medical and police personnel. The inside of the facility needs to be spacious and well lit, so that participants can see where they're going. Any sharp or electrified equipment must be stored safely, and floors must be kept clean. All equipment must be assessed to make sure no sharp edges are exposed.

STEPS IN THE COMMUNITY ORGANIZING PROCESS

- Step 1: Recognizing the issue: Needs assessment, evaluation of primary and secondary data
- Step 2: Entering the community: Interviews and observation
- Step 3: Establishing priorities and goals
- Step 4: Selecting strategies for problem-solving: Establish a tailored message
- Step 5: Implementing the plan: May be phased or total
- Step 6: Evaluating progress: Use of established indicators
- Step 7: Maintaining achievements: Continuing or discontinuing elements of the program based on evaluation

STEPS WHEN INITIATING A PLAN OF ACTION

- Step 1: Community organization: Consultation and cooperation with respected individuals and organizations in the community
- Step 2: Pretesting: Performed to acquire information about prevalent attitudes and health-related behaviors
- Step 3: Diversity training: Staff are encouraged to adjust the health communication message to the various constituents in the community
- Step 4: Effective leadership: A strong sense of organization and discipline within the health education program

NETWORKING AND COLLABORATION ROLES

Unfortunately, health educators will not always be provided with the funding and personnel to accomplish all of their goals in the manner of their choosing. Sometimes, it will be necessary to collaborate with other members of the community. For this reason, it is important for health educators to constantly be making connections, or networking, in the community. A health educator never knows when connections made in the past may yield vital resources for an ongoing health program. One of the best signs of a vital health program is a full address book.

CULTURAL COMPETENCE AND SENSITIVITY

It is important that training include an understanding of culture, cultural competence, and cultural sensitivity. Culture encompasses the ideas, beliefs, values, customs, and norms that are learned from family and community and are passed down to subsequent generations. Cultural competence entails the aptitude to understand the diversity in culture of populations and to utilize such an aptitude to ensure favorable health outcomes. Being culturally competent requires that an individual is self-aware of his or her own cultural viewpoint and his or her attitudes regarding differences and has developed cross-cultural skills. Being culturally sensitive requires understanding and respecting the beliefs of different cultures.

DEVELOPING TRAINING OBJECTIVES

When developing training objectives, it is important to understand and to use health education theories. Health education theories delineate a guide to behavior expectations. Training objectives should have a strong foundation in health education theories since these theories yield answers as to why people behave in a certain manner, what the best means are for intervention, and exactly what must be evaluated and monitored. Health education theories also enable the program planning to effectively choose strategies for the implementation of health education based upon the knowledge of behavioral influences and the ability to monitor change.

SELECTION OF TRAINING PARTICIPANTS

There are important attributes to be considered when selecting participants needed for implementation. Individuals should have a desire to educate with good communication skills. The participants to be trained will be the ones who will be delivering future interventions; therefore, it is quite important that these people have a good set of technology skills. Participants for training should have ready availability and need to comprehend the cultural or organizational context in which the intervention will be performed. When selecting a participant for training for implementation, it is also imperative that the person have the support of management.

IMPLEMENTING THE CONSTRUCTS OF SOCIAL COGNITIVE THEORY

The following are strategies in which to implement the constructs of the social cognitive theory in training: address more than one element of reciprocal determinism; engineer the environment; address individual skill-building; clarify values; understand the need to provide a great deal of practice; utilize practice repetition; enable observational learning; capitalize upon verbal persuasion; use learning in increments; provide skill-training to foster mastery in behavior; capitalize upon previous experiences; provide models of similar situations; use testimonials; foster self-awareness of the physical and the emotional responses; enable avenues to regulate and to foster self-control; and encourage the use of journaling.

IMPLEMENTING THE TTM STAGES OF CHANGE

The following are strategies in which to implement the stages of change in the TTM: increase awareness, make the risks personal, emphasize self-efficacy, aid in the development of definitive plans, establish short-term goals, give specific resources, give feedback and positive reinforcement, aid in solving problems, give opportunities for social support, aid in establishing coping strategies, provide reminders of benefits, describe the pros and the cons of change for the individual (individual consequences, consequences for others, individual reactions, and the reactions of others), establish self-awareness of behaviors that are problematic, and utilize empathy/family interventions.

HEALTH BEHAVIOR MODEL

The health behavior model is a model that is based upon value-expectancy; this model focuses upon the cognitive factors that tend to cause individual predisposition to health behavior. The health behavior model uses the premise that a person is more likely to act if he values the outcome and anticipates certain actions will achieve the outcome. The health behavior model has six constructs: perceived susceptibility, perceived severity, perceived benefits, perceived barriers, cues to action, and self-efficacy. The construct in the health behavior model that is the weakest is that of perceived seriousness.

THEORY OF REASONED ACTION/THEORY OF PLANNED BEHAVIOR

The theory of reasoned action/theory of planned behavior states, "A person's behavior is determined by intention to perform the behavior, and this intention is a function of attitude toward the behavior and subjective norm. It is an attempt to explain the relationship among attitudes, beliefs, and behavior." The theory of reasoned action has three constructs: behavioral intention, attitude, and subjective norm. The theory of reasoned action is useful in program planning and training because it serves to identify the how and where of target strategies for behavioral change. The theory of planned behavior focuses upon understanding behavioral motivations.

46

ADULT LEARNING

Adult learning is also known as andragogy. There are multiple aspects to be considered when training adults. It is important to remember that adults will be motivated to learn if they possess needs that learning will address. Adults are more oriented to learning that is applicable to life (life-centered). One should also be cognizant of the idea that experience is the best learning source. Adults are also considered to be self-directed learners. It is vital to remember to always take into account the individual differences of the adult learner. It is also necessary to engage the adult learner with explanations.

The models for adult learning are as follows: ARCS Motivation Model, Gagne's Theory of Instruction, Bloom's Taxonomy, and Maslow's Hierarchy of Needs. The ARCS Motivation Model involves the following elements: attention, relevance, confidence, and satisfaction. The ARCS model is comprised of many motivational theories. The basic purpose of the ARCS model is to give learners time and motivation to gain new knowledge. Attention refers to "capturing and maintaining interest and attention." Relevance refers to knowing the needs of the learner and giving chances to pair activities of learning to motives for learning.

GAGNE'S THEORY OF INSTRUCTION

Gagne's Theory of Instruction basically separates learning into categories. The categories include verbal information, cognitive strategies, intellectual skills, and attitudes. Gagne's Theory of Instruction gives nine events of instruction that will lead to learning. The nine events that lead to learning are: gaining attention, informing the learner of the objectives, building on prior knowledge, presenting the stimulus, providing guidance, eliciting performance, providing feedback, assessing performance, and enhancing retention and transfer. When applying Gagne's Theory, it is important to explain the importance of the training and to provide immediate feedback.

BLOOM'S TAXONOMY

Bloom's Taxonomy classifies the learning objectives that are developed and focuses on the concept that instruction needs to possess higher-ordered objectives that are felt to be intellectually demanding. The classifications in Bloom's Taxonomy include knowledge, comprehension, application, analysis, synthesis, and evaluation. The skills to be shown for knowledge are information recall and recall of the major ideas; the verbs to describe knowledge are *define*, *describe*, *label*, and *list*. The skill to be exhibited in comprehension is that of understanding the information; the verbs used to describe comprehension are *explain*, *outline*, and *summarize*.

The remaining classifications of Bloom's Taxonomy are application, analysis, synthesis, and evaluation. The skills to be shown in application include utilization of the information and the ability to solve problems while using the acquired skill. The verbs to describe application are *apply*, *construct*, *illustrate*, and *show*. The skills to be exhibited in analysis are the identification of components and the recognition of various patterns. Verbs used to describe analysis are *analyze*, *distinguish*, *compare*, and *explain*. Synthesis skills to be shown are the ability to correlate several areas of knowledge and to predict or to draw conclusions; the verbs for synthesis are *construct*, *create*, *devise*, and *formulate*. Evaluation skills are the ability to compare ideas and to choose the basis of arguments; the verbs are *assess*, *choose*, *judge*, and *justify*.

MASLOW'S HIERARCHY

Maslow's Hierarchy has the following needs: physiologic, safety, love, esteem, and self-actualization. Physiologic needs are the necessity of food, water, and warmth, and may be applied to training by providing breaks/snacks/meals. Safety refers to security and may be applied in training by providing a safe environment and by allowing questions. Love refers to the need to belong and may be addressed in training by creating positive group dynamics and acceptance. Esteem needs are status and achievement and may be met in training by recognizing achievements and positive reinforcement for learning. Self-actualization is the need for personal fulfillment and may be met by challenging the learner.

PUTTING A HEALTH EDUCATION PROGRAM INTO ACTION

In health education, there are three distinct ways of implementing a program.

- Pilot testing: Otherwise known as field testing; all elements of the program are implemented, but on a small scale; program participants must be similar to members of the target population
- Phasing in: Gradual implementation of all program elements to target population; program can be gradually applied to a larger population, a larger geographic area, or can gradually provide more services
- Total implementation: Program is implemented in its entirety to the target population from the beginning

IMPLEMENTATION PROCESS

Implementation is the process of putting a project, service, or program into effect. One seeks to set up, manage, and execute the project, service, or program. The process of implementation involves 5 phases. Phase 1 entails involving individuals or organizations that have decided to participate in an intervention or program. Phase 2 designates responsibilities and estimates resource needs. Phase 3 develops a system to manage the program. Phase 4 of the implementation process entails the actual process of going forward with plan action. Phase 5 is the sustainment or termination of the program.

PHASES OF THE IMPLEMENTATION PROCESS

The implementation of a health education program occurs in five distinct phases.

- Phase 1: The population in question is encouraged to participate in the program; this phase emphasizes the importance of having adequate staff and a willing target population for a successful program
- Phase 2: Resource and task inventory; it is absolutely essential to have a precise understanding of the resources and manpower that will be required to implement a program; also, the inventory needs to include a description of the sources of resources and manpower
- Phase 3: A system for overseeing the program is established; it must include clear indicators and a well-defined timetable
- Phase 4: Implementation; may be total or partial
- Phase 5: Program assessment, with special attention to the established indicators

SCENARIO ONE

You are implementing a health education program that involves setting up a free community health fair.

Identify which method of putting a program into action would be most appropriate.

A free community health fair is likely to be a one-time event in which members of the target community can receive complementary information and supplies. It would not make sense to only provide part of the total available resources at a free community health fair. For this reason, total implementation of the program plan is the only acceptable method in this case. Total implementation is always the best option for health programs that are very specific in duration and intent. If there were to be a series of health affairs, it might be appropriate to gradually increase or adjust the available materials depending on the interest of the target community. For a one-time event, though, total implementation is the only reasonable option.

SCENARIO TWO

You are planning a birth control education program in a rural community where there is a high rate of teenage pregnancy.

1. Describe how you would start the implementation process for such a program.

   If you are planning to implement a birth control education program in a rural community, you would begin by obtaining as much information as possible about the members of that community. You would conduct interviews with local residents and peruse all available records for useful information. You would then take whatever steps possible to encourage interest among the target population. This can be done by enlisting the aid of local leaders, like politicians and religious figures, or by placing advertisements in the local press. In a small community, it would also be important for you to establish personal relationships and cultivate a good rapport with the young people.

2. You have gained acceptance for the program. Describe the next step in the implementation process.

   After laying the foundations for community interest in your health education program, you would need to perform a comprehensive inventory of the resources and tasks required to successfully complete the program. You might want to lead sex education classes, disseminate information about birth control, and conduct private conferences with at-risk youths. You'll probably need educational literature, models, and sample birth control. You may need volunteers from the community. Above all, you certainly will need money. After you have completed your inventory, you need to determine where all of this equipment and aid will come from.

3. You have gained acceptance for the program and have identified the necessary tasks and resources. Describe the next step in the implementation process.

   After you have performed a comprehensive resource and task inventory, you need to develop your plan of implementation. In order to be effective, you need to make sure that your methodology is appropriate for the target population. Literature and visual presentations should not be too sophisticated for the members of the population to understand. All educational activities should be conducted in a location that is accessible to the relevant members of the community. The resources required for the implementation of the program should not put undue strain on finances or manpower.

4. You have gained acceptance for the program and have identified the necessary tasks and resources. You have planned the program activities. Describe the next step in the implementation process.

   After you have determined the appropriate resources and activities for the implementation of your health education program, you can begin to outline the sequence in which program components will be implemented. In order to achieve the goals of the program in a certain amount of time, you need to set short-term goals for the accomplishment of program objectives. You also need to establish a set of objectives that will result in the achievement of long-term goals. For instance, in order to achieve the goal of increasing birth control awareness, you might set as an objective holding monthly awareness meetings with local students.

5. You are ready to put the plan into action. Identify which method you would use and explain why.

   After you have completed a detailed outline and timeline of the tasks and resources to be required by the health education program, you can begin to implement your plan. You may decide to implement the entire plan at once, or you may decide to implement some parts earlier than others. In a wide ranging and multifaceted campaign like a birth control education program, it might be a good idea to introduce some aspects of the program and then make useful adjustments to the other parts. Another way to phase in a program of this nature is to offer it to a limited section of the community before expanding it to include the entire community.

PRE-TESTING LEARNERS BEFORE BEGINNING A COMMUNITY EDUCATION INITIATIVE

Health educators will often elect to perform pretesting in a community before establishing a comprehensive program plan. Pretesting is done to measure the pre-existing knowledge, skills, and attitudes of the target population. Many health educators believe that pretesting enables them to develop more sophisticated and appropriate strategies for health education. In any case, it is useful for setting expectations and reasonable goals for a program. Of course, if pretesting is performed before a plan has been fully established, it may not effectively measure the eventual program goals. Also, pretesting does little to suggest the potential for the success of a health education program

SCENARIO TWO CONTINUED

You are planning a birth control education program in a rural community where there is a high rate of teenage pregnancy.

Explain how you would use pre-testing as an aid to the implementation process.

If you are establishing a birth control education program in a rural community, you would probably want to pre-test small groups of the community before totally implementing your program. In this sort of situation, pre-testing would give you an idea of the knowledge base and prevailing attitudes of members of the community. With this information, you could adapt your program to better serve the needs of the community. You might find, for instance, that many members of the community are opposed to birth control for religious reasons. Obviously, this would affect your subsequent presentations.

AID GIVEN BY THEORIES WHEN HEALTH EDUCATORS ARE PLANNING PROGRAMS

Health educators should have a theoretical grounding to help inform their program plans. The theories of behavior are the most pertinent to a health educator, because they include prescriptions for positively altering health-related behaviors. These theoretical perspectives on health behavior can help educators to develop a comprehensive program for improving health-related behavior. Some health educators are partial towards one particular theory of health behavior, while other

50

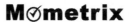

educators treat the theoretical canon as a buffet, picking and choosing those elements which are helpful to the task at hand.

SOCIAL COGNITIVE THEORY

The social cognitive theory of behavior asserts that individuals learn to behave in certain ways depending on the motivations and inhibitions in their environment. An individual will have his or her own predisposition, and behavior will derive from the interplay between disposition and the environment. According to the social cognitive theory, the best way to encourage positive changes in behavior is to increase the individual's feeling of self-efficacy, or the ability to make positive changes. In other words, making changes in the individual's predisposition can overcome inhibitions stemming from the environment.

According to the Social Cognitive Theory of learning, behavior is determined by personal characteristics, and the environment in which the behavior occurs, and the nature of the behavior. The ways in which these three elements influence one another is referred to as Reciprocal Determinism. Health professionals who seek to change behavior, therefore, will need to influence all three of these factors in order to achieve permanent improvement. Specifically, health professionals seek to cultivate a sense of self efficacy in the individual; in other words, they seek to show the individual that improvement is possible. A health professional will also concentrate on giving the individual the knowledge and skills to change his or her behavior, and will try to instill confidence that using the new behavioral patterns will create a desired outcome.

TECHNIQUES FOR BRINGING ABOUT A CHANGE IN BEHAVIOR

Remember that Social Cognitive Theory insists that changes must be made to the individual, the behavior, and the environment. So, the techniques used to implement this theory must treat each of these three areas. The individual must be provided with education about the causes and consequences of his or her behavior. He or she must be taught new patterns of behavior to replace old pathologies. The individual must make changes to his or her environment, whether this means altering his or her home or avoiding problematic situations. In any case, the health educator needs to impress upon the individual that behavioral change will only occur when specific steps are made to change the environment and attitude.

RECIPROCAL DETERMINISM

Reciprocal Determinism is a concept found in Social Cognitive Theory that states that individual characteristics, behavior characteristics, and behavior environment are all intertwined. In order to achieve a permanent change in behavior, all three of these elements need to be positively adjusted. To this end, individuals need to develop a feeling of self-efficacy, the knowledge and skills to perform new patterns of behavior, and a positive expectation for the implementation of the new behavior patterns. Dependence on the concept of Reciprocal Determinism is one reason why health education programs always include both learning and behavior objectives.

TRANSTHEORETICAL MODEL

The transtheoretical model of behavior change describes how individuals can develop new and positive habits. Specifically, it offers reasons for why some behavior changes are permanent while others are only temporary. The Transtheoretical model outlines six stages in behavior change: precontemplation, contemplation, preparation/commitment, action, maintenance, and termination. Perhaps the most important insight of this model is that behavior change is not an instantaneous event, but rather a process that unfolds in distinct phases.

The Transtheoretical Model of behavior outlines six distinct stages of behavior change. Each of these stages of change requires a different kind of intervention on the part of the health professional. The stages of change are as follows:

- Precontemplation: Individual does not recognize a problem
- Contemplation: Individual acknowledges a problem but is not yet ready to change
- Preparation/commitment: individual decides to change and begins to assemble relevant information
- Action: Individual begins to change behavior
- Maintenance: Individual avoids recidivism, in part by recognizing the benefits of the new behavior
- Termination: New behavior is fully learned and habitual; almost no risk of recidivism

HEALTH BELIEF MODEL

The Health Belief Model of behavior change states that when individuals acquire more information about a health problem, they are more likely to change their behavior. When individuals consider a particular health problem, there are six core beliefs that exert influence on their behavior. First, the individual must believe that he or she could potentially be affected by the health problem. Second, the individual must believe that the health problem is a significant threat. Third, the individual must believe that the benefits of preventive behavior are greater than the costs associated. Fourth, the individual must believe that he or she is capable of changing his or her behavior. Fifth, the individual must be encouraged to change behavior. Sixth, the individual must believe that he or she will be able to perform the new behavior.

The health belief model for behavior change seeks to explain why individuals perform certain health-related behaviors rather than others. Specifically, this model points to four primary factors as being directly related to health behavior. First, an individual has to believe that his or her health may be in jeopardy as the result of a given behavior. Second, the individual has to understand how an adverse health condition may result in pain, financial problems, or other negative consequences. Third, the individual must believe that the benefits of the behavior change outweigh the negative consequences of the current behavior pattern. Fourth, the person must receive some direct cue that spurs him or her to action.

THEORY OF PLANNED BEHAVIOR

The Theory of Planned Behavior (TPB) declares that the primary factor in behavior change is simply the intention to make the change. This theory is similar to the theory of reasoned action, but it also includes perceived behavioral control as an influence on intention. In other words, individuals will be more likely to decide to perform an activity if they believe they can control it. Other factors that contribute to intention are attitude and subjective norm (a positive belief about the behavior in question).

The theory of planned behavior emphasizes the varying degrees of control that an individual will have over his or her behavior or attitude. This theory is especially concerned with assessing how much perceived control an individual has. If an individual feels that he or she has no control over his or her behavior, changes are unlikely. On the other hand, an increased feeling of self efficacy leads to health improvements. According to this model, it is the job of a health educator to show the client that he or she has more control over health behavior and consequences.

DIFFUSION OF INNOVATION THEORY

The diffusion of innovation theory describes the way in which a new idea or product is distributed throughout a marketplace. In health education, this theory is applied to describe the way new patterns of behavior spread throughout a community. Research indicates that new behavior patterns and innovations in health activity are typically adopted at first only by a few educated members of the community. Over time, however, advances in health behavior that yield positive results will be adopted by more and more members of the community. The diffusion of innovation theory outlines the five stages for the diffusion of innovation: knowledge, persuasion, decision, implementation, and confirmation.

The Diffusion of Innovation theory considers the ways in which new ideas or practices are gradually accepted by society. There are five identifiable stages of adoption:

- Awareness: Individuals or communities are introduced to the innovation
- Interest (information): Individuals or communities endeavor to find out more about the innovation
- Evaluation: Individuals or communities consider the consequences of the innovation and decide whether or not to give it a try
- Trial: Individuals or communities use the innovation
- Adoption: Individuals or communities elect to continue using the innovation

According to the Diffusion of Innovation theory, new ideas and practices gradually spread throughout a society. The speed and pervasiveness with which innovation will spread through a society is determined by the characteristics of the target population. According to this theory, there are five types of innovation adopters:

- Innovators: Individuals who are open to new ideas, and are the first to accept and utilize the innovation
- Early adopters: Among the first to adopt innovation; often individuals whose behavior is emulated by others
- Early majority: Individuals who take their time before deciding to accept innovation
- Late majority: Individuals who take even longer than the early majority, and sometimes only accept innovation after it becomes necessary
- Laggards: Individuals who continue to resist innovation

PROMOTING CULTURAL SENSITIVITY

Health educators are likely to be working with individuals from distinct cultural backgrounds, and so need to develop cultural sensitivity. This means avoiding value judgments based on culture, and respecting the beliefs and traditions of each individual. In some cases, you may find that an individual's culture prevents him or her from receiving all the benefits of the health education program. When this occurs, you must remain patient and seek alternative methods of instruction that can minimize this problem. As much as possible, you should partner with members of the multicultural community. Also, clients of the health education program should not be allowed to express negative opinions of the culture and heritage of others.

ENSURING PROGRAMS ARE CULTURALLY AND DEMOGRAPHICALLY SENSITIVE

When constructing health programs, educators need to be culturally and demographically sensitive to the members of the community. Certain health issues, particularly sexual matters, may be controversial in a community; health educators should seek out methods of instruction that do not alienate traditional beliefs. When unsure, health educators should consult a respected member of the community. As much as possible, health educators should strive to tailor their methods and message to the demographic and cultural background of the audience.

INSTRUCTIONAL TECHNOLOGY SKILLS

More and more, health educators are required to incorporate instructional technology into their lessons. Some of the basic instructional technology with which a health educator must be familiar is PowerPoint, e-mail, and basic search engines. In order to obtain the most current research data, health educators will need to know how to access the major databases online. In the interest of presenting information in a variety of media, health educators also need to be familiar with video and audio equipment. Some health educators find it useful to create their own websites, in which case they will need to become familiar with site design and maintenance.

ACTING AS GROUP FACILITATORS

Insofar as they will need to assess group dynamics and improve the performance of a group, health educators can be described as group facilitators. In some cases, health educators will be directly leading a group of students, while in other cases the health educator will serve merely as a guide. One of the best ways to encourage positive group dynamics is to make explicit the intention and organization of the program. When individuals understand their own roles and responsibilities, they are more likely to avoid conflict.

FACILITATING CHANGE IN HEALTH BEHAVIORS

Health educators will need to choose the implementation strategy that is most appropriate for the health program and target population. Small, single-pointed programs may be implemented all at once, but larger, multipart programs may benefit from a phased or partial implementation. In a phased implementation, only selected parts of the program are implemented at first. In a partial implementation, all phases of the program are implemented on a section of the community. Finally, the implementation strategy that is most appropriate will depend on whether the health program is using primary, secondary, or tertiary prevention methods.

MONITORING IMPLEMENTATION

The Gantt method, Program Evaluation and Review Technique (PERT), and Critical Path Method (CPM) are means by which implementation of health education may be monitored. The Gantt method helps to monitor health education implementation by illustrating a timeline that shows important activities and outputs that are considered important identifiers of the implementation process. Program Evaluation and Review Technique is used to generate an illustration to facilitate scheduling and to show the project timeline or the project management plan. The Critical Path Method also is used to illustrate the schedule and to show the timeline or management plan

The **steps** needed to ensure a plan is implemented consistently include:

- Build support for the plan: Involve key stakeholders in generating support. Keep people informed about progress while developing the plan and outline benefits of the plan.
- Develop a plan for implementation: Outline the steps to implementation and the expected timeline in detail using the best estimates.
- Train those guiding implementation so that their approaches are consistent.
- Carry out pilot programs or small tests of change, if possible, in order to identify problems and make corrections before full implementation.
- Assess each step in the implementation: Monitor continuously and make adjustments as needed. Seek out feedback from staff and participants in the program being implemented.

- Promote: Report early successes, maintain a dashboard to provide updates, reward participants and key supporters, provide information to media, and discuss the program one-on-one and in team and group meetings.

IMPLEMENTATION MAY VARY DEPENDING ON DIFFERENT SETTINGS

Health educators function in a variety of different settings, so they will need to use various implementation methods depending on circumstances. When working in a business, for instance, health educators can count on having a "captive audience" and full institutional support for their efforts. In a community, on the other hand, health educators will need to take more strenuous efforts to encourage the interest of the population. When working in schools, health educators will need to tailor their methods to the particular abilities and attitudes of the students. In a college or university, educators will be able to assume a greater degree of knowledge on the part of their clients and can focus on refining positive health behaviors.

STAGES OF CHANGE IN THE TRANSTHEORETICAL MODEL

- precontemplation: individual must be made aware of the necessity of change
- contemplation: individual should be encouraged to seek out specific plans for change
- preparation/commitment: individual should be setting goals, and considering the benefits of behavior change
- action: individual should be given feedback and encouragement as plan of behavior change is implemented
- maintenance: individual should be prevented from relapse and given further support
- termination: individual should know that support is available if necessary

IMPLEMENTING A HEALTH EDUCATION PROGRAM TERMS

- Coalition: an assemblage of individuals and organizations from different backgrounds but with a common purpose; typically, the members of a coalition are given different roles and tasks depending on their areas of expertise
- Culture: the agreed-upon ethics and interests of a coalition or group of people unified by a common purpose
- Strategic planning: the laying out of a series of tasks and objectives which will ultimately result in the achievement of long-term goals

Conduct Evaluation and Research Related to Health Education/Promotion

EVALUATION AND RESEARCH

In health education, evaluation is the process of measuring the degree to which a program meets the objectives for which it was designed. In order to be effective, evaluation should be an ongoing process. The methods of evaluation, known as indicators, should be specific and explicit in the objectives of the program. Evaluation is not meant to be a punishment for employees; rather, it is an opportunity for them to improve their performance. In many cases, the supplier of financial aid to a health education program will want constant evaluation to make sure that money is being spent effectively.

In order to be an effective health educator, you need to be skilled at evaluation and research. Effective evaluation requires the establishment and use of appropriate indicators, as well as the subjective apparatus to make judgments when objective indicators are not possible. Health educators also need to be able to compare data from their own program with the results of other similar programs, in order to make decisions for continuation or termination of a program. As for research, health educators need to be familiar with the most current work that is being done in their particular field. There are a myriad of sources for health education information on the Internet; health educators need to be able to assess the reliability of this information.

Health educators should have a variety of evaluation strategies in their repertoire. The most important thing is that evaluation is always done in accordance with the indicators established during the planning phase. A number of systems have been developed to organize evaluation. The decision-making model, for instance, evaluates the criteria that are used for making administrative decisions in the program. In some cases, health educators will need to use subjective means such as interviews and observation to assess the quality of the program. At other times, it will be possible to assemble a body of numerical data.

WAYS IN WHICH EVALUATION CAN BE USED IN DIFFERENT PRACTICE SETTINGS

A well-trained health educator will need to use his or her evaluation skills in a number of different situations. Evaluation is not just about assessing the progress of one's own program; a health educator will also need to evaluate the available literature on a particular health subject so that they can make an accurate and comprehensive presentation to the members of the community. In order to compile a proper needs assessment, a health educator will have to evaluate primary and secondary data, as well as observations and interviews. Once a program has been implemented, a health educator will have to evaluate its progress in the light of the established indicators.

RELIABILITY VS. VALIDITY

Two of the terms that health educators use frequently when evaluating a program are reliability and validity. Reliability is the degree to which a program is likely to achieve similar results when implemented in similar conditions. Reliable programs can be repeated with a great deal of confidence. Validity, on the other hand, is the degree to which an instrument of measurement is applied to the appropriate object. For instance, a smoking cessation program might use as a valid indicator the improvement and cardiovascular fitness; it would not be appropriate, however, to use weight loss as a valid indicator.

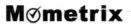

CREATING A PURPOSE STATEMENT

A purpose statement is defined as a tool to identify what is to be learned from the evaluation and the research and serves to focus and steer the collection and analysis of data. A mission statement may also be considered a purpose statement and is a statement of the distinctive purpose of and unique reason for the existence of a program. It can be a one-sentence statement of a short narrative that broadly defines the program's purpose. This statement is used to identify the scope or focus of the organization or program.

DEVELOPING EVALUATION/RESEARCH QUESTIONS

Evaluation questions are designed to designate boundaries for an evaluation by determining what areas of the program are to be the focuses. It is important to consider indicators when developing evaluation questions. An indicator is information or statistics that provide evidence of progress toward outcomes. A baseline indicator is the value of the indicator prior to implementation. A target indicator is the expected value of an indicator at a specific point in time. Indicators should be created from a logic model and typically have five characteristics of credibility.

GUIDING THE EVALUATION PROCESS

It is important to use process evaluation questions to enable understanding of the internal and the external forces that can impact the activities of the program. Process evaluation may involve combinations of different measures that may be taken as a program is implemented to maintain or to improve the quality and standards of the program performance or delivery. The process evaluation may also serve as documentation of the provisions of the program to individuals and the success of the program's provision. The process evaluation typically measures the ways in which changes were generated.

DATA ANALYSIS PLAN

The design of the evaluation needs to be specific and designate data collection (when it is collected and from whom). When choosing an evaluation design, the following need to be addressed: limitations to time and finances, current political climate, number of participants, data type (qualitative data, quantitative data, both forms of data), data analysis methods and skills, and access to a group to use for comparative purposes. To facilitate an evaluation design and data analysis, comparison and evaluation groups should be similar, pre- and post- data measurements should be taken, and issues with internal and external validity should be minimized.

IDENTIFYING USEABLE QUESTIONS FROM EXISTING INSTRUMENTS

The following evaluation models may be used to identify useable questions from existing instruments: attainment model, decision-making model, goal-free model, naturalistic model, systems analysis model, and utilization-focused model. The attainment model uses evaluation standards and instruments that primarily target the objectives and goals of the program. The decision-making model uses instruments that focus upon the elements that yield context, input, processes, and products to use when making decisions. The goal-free model has instruments that provide all outcomes (including unintentional positive or negative outcomes). The systems analysis model uses instruments that serve to quantify the program's effects.

CREDIBLE INDICATORS

There are five characteristics of credible indicators. The five characteristics are clearly linked to intervention outcome; given in specific, measurable terms; appropriate for the population being served; feasible given data collection resources and skills; and valid and reliable to stakeholders. The following are examples of evidence sources for program indicators: survey questions, intake questions from clients, staff logs or records from the organization, demonstration of skills, and direct observations. It is important to remember that indicators may be changed, modified, or even established during the course of the evaluation. Evidence sources for program indicators need to be specific.

DEVELOPING VALID, RELIABLE EVALUATION INSTRUMENTS

In order to obtain reliable data, health educators need to have reliable instruments of data collection. The appropriate instrument of data collection will depend on the intent of the program, the intent of the evaluation, and the information being acquired. Focus groups, for example, are a good way of obtaining information about the prevailing attitudes on a health-related issue in a given community. It is important that the data collection instruments limit themselves to obtaining information directly related to the health education program in question; collection instruments that obtain too much information will be as unhelpful as those that obtain too little.

SELECTING DATA COLLECTION METHODS APPROPRIATE FOR MEASURING OBJECTIVES OF A STUDY

The ideal data collection methods will specifically target the most important elements of the study, those that most clearly prove or disprove the hypothesis. It is also important that the data collection methods be appropriate to the scale of the study, meaning that they do not cost too much money or require too much time. For example, for a small-scale study it would not be effective to conduct one-on-one interviews with every member of a large population. On the other hand, if a survey requires information from every member of the target community, it will be ineffective to use mailing surveys as the instruments of data collection.

IRB (INSTITUTIONAL REVIEW BOARD)

In health research, the initials IRB stand for Institutional Review Board. This group serves as a general supervisor of health research. One of the tasks of the board is to make sure that research subjects are treated with respect and care. Another task is to approve proposals for future research. Basically, the IRB safeguards the interests of health researchers and subjects alike. The IRB tries to prevent researchers from being blindsided by accusations of negligence or liability.

APPLYING ETHICAL STANDARDS WHEN DEVELOPING AN EVALUATION OR RESEARCH PLAN

The ethical standards to be applied when developing an evaluation or research plan include respect for autonomy, promotion of social justice, active promotion of good, and avoidance of harm. Since health education evaluations or research often involve the use of human subjects, it is imperative to devise an evaluation or research plan that protects the privacy of the participants involved. Data that is collected for research or for evaluation must be stored, utilized, and disclosed in such a manner as to protect the privacy of the participants.

IMPLEMENTING A RESEARCH PLAN

When implementing a research plan, the first objective is to gauge the scale of the project. Later decisions regarding research design and data analysis will depend on an accurate assessment of the project scale. As the research plan is revised, educators must remain conscious of preserving internal and external validity. A project with internal validity is not affected by things outside of its purview. A project with external validity can be applied to other, related programs when it is complete.

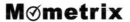

SECTIONS OF RESEARCH REPORTS

There are five important sections in any research report compiled by a health educator:

- Introduction: Outlines the basic intent and methodology of the research
- Literature review: Summarizes all of the professional literature that was used as background for the research
- Methodology: Summary of the research techniques used, including all instruments of data collection
- Results: Assembled data in accordance with prescribed indicators
- Conclusions/recommendations/summary: Evaluates the results, assesses the pros and cons of the research methodology, and suggests possible implications of the research

ACADEMIC LITERATURE

EVALUATING RESEARCH RESULTS FOUND IN ACADEMIC LITERATURE

Health educators will need to keep a number of things in mind when evaluating academic research for use in a health education program. The overall concern is to be sure that the research is applicable to the health education program in question. In order to determine this, the health educator will need to pay particular attention to the stated purpose, hypothesis, and research design of the study. Sometimes, research which seems to be similar to a given health program will turn out to have been conducted in conditions that make it irrelevant. A health educator also needs to pay attention to which instruments were used to collect data during the research, and how the collected data was organized.

SYNTHESIZING INFORMATION FOUND IN THE LITERATURE

There is such a huge amount of health literature available these days, it has become even more important for a health educator to be able to organize and synthesize this information before presenting it to the general public. A great deal of research is ongoing in health-related matters; a health educator needs to be able to determine which research is relevant and how it applies to his or her health program. At all times, the health educator needs to keep in mind the level of education and prevailing attitudes of the target audience, so as to disseminate information that will be engaging and useful.

RESEARCH METHODS

The research methods used by health educators are typically described as either qualitative or quantitative. Qualitative research is more subjective and focused on the accumulation of subjective information. Interviews and observation are two common sources of qualitative research. In order to obtain consistent and useful qualitative data, researchers need to be trained thoroughly. Quantitative research, on the other hand, is performed using accepted and standardized systems of measurement. Quantitative research is easier to analyze and organize mathematically. Most scientific research is quantitative, though it may stem from qualitative observations.

DATA COLLECTION METHODS

There are numerous methods by which to collect data. Methods may include written surveys, personal interviews, indirect and direct observation, case studies, individual and group assessments, role playing, peer reviews, testimonials, debriefing activities, and activity logs. An impact evaluation measures the knowledge, skills, attitudes, and beliefs of the participant. There are five methods by which to collect impact evaluation data: pre-test/post-test, participant demonstration, participant role-playing, participation observation, and participant interviews.

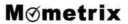

TEST VALIDITY

Validity is the degree to which a test or assessment measures what it is intended to measure. Internal validity is the degree to which the program caused the change that was measured; were changes in participants due to program or chance? Some of the threats to internal validity include history, mortality, maturation, testing, selection, and diffusion/imitation of treatment. Threats to internal validity may be mediated by randomization of selection of the participants and assignment of the participants. Internal validity is important in monitoring the process and in monitoring the outcomes.

> **Review Video: Testing Validity**
> Visit mometrix.com/academy and enter code: 315457

MEASUREMENT VALIDITY

Measurement validity is the degree to which an instrument measures what the evaluator wants it to measure. Measurement validity consists of the following types: face, content, criterion, and construct. Face validity is the extent to which an instrument appears to be measuring what it is supposed to measure. Content validity is the extent to which an instrument samples items from the content desired. Criterion validity is the extent to which an instrument correlates with another measure of a variable. Construct validity is the extent to which the concepts of an instrument relate to the concepts of a particular theory.

EXTERNAL VALIDITY

External validity is the generalizability of the results beyond the participants; if we do this again with a different group, will we get the same results. The threats to external validity include the following: social desirability, expectancy effect, Hawthorne effect, and placebo effect. The social desirability threat occurs when the participant tries to respond in a manner that they think that the evaluator desires. The expectancy effect is also called a self-fulfilling prophecy/Rosenthal effect and reflects the idea that expectations placed upon people cause them to act as expected. The Hawthorne effect is a change in behavior from feeling special. Placebo effect is a behavior change due to belief in treatment effectiveness.

DESCRIPTIVE STATISTICS

Descriptive statistics are utilized to describe data and to decrease a large quantity of data into a few elemental measurements that entirely describe data distribution. Frequency is the total number of observations within a category. Mean is the average, relative center of a normally distributed (bell-shaped) distribution. Median is the number that is in the center of an ordered data set. The mode is the number that occurs most often in a data set. Descriptive statistics serve to yield simple summaries regarding the sample and the measures. Descriptive statistics provide a means of quantitative data analysis when combined with simple graphics analysis.

INFERENTIAL STATISTICS

Inferential statistics are a procedural system used to obtain conclusions from sets of data that come from systems that are impacted by random variation. Data derived from inferential statistics are used to formulate judgments or inferences about a population. Nominal data are mutually exclusive exhaustive data. Ordinal data are mutually exclusive exhaustive ordered data, in which the distance between categories cannot be measured. Interval data are mutually exclusive exhaustive ordered data, in which the distance between categories can be measured but with no absolute 0. Ratio data are mutually exclusive exhaustive ordered data, in which the distance between categories can be measured with absolute 0.

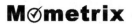

DEVELOPING AND EVALUATING DATA-GATHERING INSTRUMENTS AND PROCESSES

When developing instruments of data collection, it is important to ensure that they will be used in a regular and well defined manner. For instance, the results of interviews will not be useful if the interviews are not conducted in a consistent way. For this reason, it is important that all those members of staff who will be conducting interviews be trained. The leaders of the health education program should also work to make sure that data collection instruments will not obtain too much information, thus requiring a great deal of time to be spent winnowing out the inessential data from the essential.

The general concern that health educators should have about the instruments used to gather data in a research project is that they be appropriate to the stated goals of the research. For instance, some health projects will use interviews and surveys to collect data for analysis. This is appropriate for obtaining information about changes in attitude or perception, but does not provide the sort of objective, hard data that may be required to prove a hypothesis. A precise measurement of weight loss in a given individual, for instance, is more easily obtained on a scale than through a written survey.

LAWS AND REGULATIONS ASSOCIATED WITH THE MANAGEMENT OF PARTICIPANT DATA

The Health Insurance Portability and Accountability Act (HIPAA) establishes federal regulations for protection of the privacy of **participant data** if it is derived from patients. The privacy rule protects all information in health records as well as billing information and conversations among individuals and healthcare providers. The security rule establishes rules for safeguarding information. Additionally, states often have laws related to privacy and security of data. Research involving human subjects may require review by the Institutional Review Board with guidance provided by the Code of Federal Regulations (Title 45, part 46) When collecting data, the original data forms should be stored as well as data in electronic devices. There are few regulations about the length of time data must be stored, but most regulations suggest 5 to 10 years. There are also few regulations that deal directly with data collection and storage with the exception of information stored in electronic health records. The organization should establish a policy for storage of research data.

ANALYZING AFTER AN EVALUATION

Obviously, the most important information that data can provide is whether a program is succeeding or failing. This judgment is based on the degree to which the program is able to meet its objectives and goals. An evaluation that generates a great deal of information about all aspects of the program will be more helpful, as it will allow health educators to fine tune the program by adjusting some elements and keeping others consistent. The quality of evaluation data may lead educators to subsequently adjust the indicators that are used to diagnose problems within the program.

RESEARCH DATA

Research data is simply the performance of the program according to the indicators originally set out. Most of the time, it will center on progress or the lack thereof within the target population, specifically the degree to which the target population makes the prescribed positive health-related behavior changes. Other data, however, will center on the administrative performance of the program. This will allow educators to determine when bureaucratic inefficiencies are preventing a program from functioning at a high level. Health educators are often required to streamline their administrative operations after evaluations indicate significant inefficiencies.

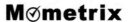

DATA ANALYSIS PLAN

It is important to have a solid data analysis plan to enable data collection in an integrated and organized fashion to facilitate data understanding and utilization. The data analysis plan should be designed to decrease data, synthesize collected data, and organize and summarize data to facilitate understanding. Existing instruments for data collection may be used but need cautious review to ensure that extraneous aspects are eliminated. It is also important to do pilot testing of existing data collection instruments.

INTERPRETING AND REPORTING THE RESULTS OF AN EVALUATION

The final stage of the evaluation process is compilation and report. In the case of quantitative study, health educators can compile data into a table for analysis. In order to do this effectively, the educator will have to be familiar with basic concepts of statistics: range, standard deviation, and dispersion. The analysis of data should also be expressed in a written document. This document should include a recommendation as to whether the program should be terminated or continued. The composition of this evaluation document should reflect its intended audience; non-experts should not be exposed to a laborious description of professional practice.

QUANTITATIVE EVALUATION VS. QUALITATIVE EVALUATION

Health educators must know the difference between quantitative and qualitative evaluation. A quantitative evaluation assembles a mass of numerical data for analysis. The frequencies of a certain behavior, scores of participants on standardized tests, the results of medical tests: these are all possible sources of numerical data for a quantitative evaluation. One advantage of quantitative evaluation is that results can be easily compared to data from another program. A qualitative evaluation, meanwhile, is a more subjective assessment of the success of the program. In some cases, it is impossible to define performance with numbers and hard data; health educators will need to use their judgment to evaluate the program. Interviews, written surveys, and direct observation are three common ways of assembling information for a qualitative evaluation.

QUESTIONS THAT NEED TO BE ADDRESSED WHEN EVALUATING RESEARCH

When evaluating research in order to synthesize data, it is important to consider several questions, including: Was the purpose of the study stated? Was the research question/hypothesis stated? Were subjects and their recruitment described? Was the design and the location described? Were data collection instruments described? Did the results reflect the research question/hypothesis? Were conclusions reflective of the research design and the data analysis? Were the implications meaningful to the priority population? When evaluating research data, it is important to distinguish between meta-analysis and pooled analysis as well.

COMPARING EVALUATION RESULTS TO OTHER FINDINGS

One of the reasons why it is important for the research design to maintain an external validity is so that evaluation results can be compared to pre-existing professional standards. There are a number of health education databases that compile records from previous programs, with the specific intention of making these records available to ongoing programs. In some cases, it may be necessary for health educators to convert one of the other sets of data so that they may be compared. For instance, it may be useful to place both sets of data on a spreadsheet using the same units of measurement.

EXPLANATIONS AND POSSIBLE LIMITATIONS OF FINDINGS

When explaining findings, conclusions need to be justified. The following need to be considered when proposing possible explanations of findings: standards, analysis, synthesis, interpretation, judgments, and recommendations. Evaluation findings are justified when they are linked to the evidence gathered and judged against agreed-upon values or standards set by the stakeholders. The standards are the values of the stakeholders. Analysis and synthesis involve the process of isolating significant results and integrating the information sources to achieve a greater understanding. Interpretation encompasses understanding the results and the evidence that has been gathered in the process.

There are numerous factors that may cause possible limitations of findings. It is important to carefully examine and analyze data to look for patterns, recurring themes, similarities, and differences. The ways in which patterns or a lack of patterns justify or do not justify answers to the evaluation questions need to be addressed. Any deviations from established patterns must be carefully studied to provide possible reasons for finding limitations. It is also pertinent to study how patterns are either supported or negated by previous studies or evaluations. Limitations of the findings may also serve to suggest that more data are needed.

REPORTING THE EFFECTIVENESS OF COMPLETED PROGRAMS

There are a few different ways for a researcher to make public the results of a program. The most common forum is a professional journal article. These articles have a prescribed format, beginning with a summary of the research goals, followed by a survey of the previous work in the research domain. The author will then describe in depth the methodology and conditions under which the research was performed. Finally, the article will report the findings of the research, including any implications or conclusions that can be drawn from the results.

COMMUNICATING FINDINGS TO STAKEHOLDERS

In preparation to utilize the evaluation results, it is important to give the primary users hypothetical results and question them as to what conclusions or decisions they would choose from reviewing the results. It is necessary to conduct periodic and interim meetings with the stakeholders to disseminate findings and possible interpretations of the results, and to draft various reports. To facilitate utilization of the findings, it is critical to address the following parameters: study design, preparation, possible feedback, careful follow-through, information distribution, and possible further uses of the information.

DISSEMINATING FINDINGS

When preparing to disseminate findings, a formal report is not necessary, but it is important to consider the audience. An effective evaluation report needs to include the following aspects: timely provision of the report, an effective summary, detailed summary of how the stakeholders were involved, and a list of the strengths and limitations/weaknesses of the findings. It should utilize vignettes, illustrations, and various examples and stories. The following are the elements of the report: introduction (executive summary, study background, problems that were addressed), literature review, methodology, results, and conclusions.

APPLICATION OF EVALUATION FINDINGS IN POLICY ANALYSIS AND PROGRAM DEVELOPMENT

When applying the evaluation findings for policy analysis or program development, it is important to do thorough implementation documentation. The documentation of implementation entails the following elements: summary of activities and of the processes of the program. An implementation evaluation is also essential and is a retrospective determination of whether the program was implemented as designed. A summative evaluation is also useful in the application of the findings of the evaluation when considering policy analysis or program development. Such an evaluation will aid decision makers in ascertaining the merits of the program.

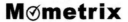

DETERMINING EFFECTIVENESS A HEALTH EDUCATION PROGRAM TERMS

- evaluation: measuring the degree to which a health education program accomplishes its intended goals; performed according to predetermined indicators
- research: the means of gathering information about health-related attitudes, behaviors, and environments
- variables: the things that are measured in an experiment; as much as possible, the variables in an experiment should be isolated and examined individually
- validity: the degree to which an experiment or study measures what it intended to measure

Administer and Manage Health Education/Promotion

GRANT PROPOSALS

Obtaining a grant is one way of ensuring fiscal resources. A grant proposal needs to include the following aspects: title page, abstract/executive summary, table of contents, introduction, background, proposed program description, resources, references, personnel and budget. The abstract is simply the summary of the program proposal. The introduction should include a detailed description of the health problem and its scope, as well as the purpose of the request for fiscal funding. The background aspect of the grant proposal is designed to provide justification for the grant and should include a literature review.

The proposed program description of a grant proposal needs to include the following aspects: goals, objectives, activities, evaluation plan, and a timeline for meeting objectives and activities. The resources section of a grant proposal details what resources are necessary such as staffing, location, etc. The reference section of a grant proposal will list any sources that were cited. The personnel section will provide resumes and job descriptions of the personnel to be involved.

BUDGET

A budget serves as a working document that aids the organization in effectively operating and evaluating the proper use of funds. The following elements will need to be addressed when preparing a budget: the way in which the organization views the program, the ways in which recent budgets and the program have been utilized, current analysis of the outcomes of the program, information and input from personnel, and possible future budget changes that may be necessary. It is essential to prepare budget reports that are to be distributed monthly, quarterly, or annually.

BUDGET REPORTS, COST ANALYSIS, AND COST-EFFECTIVENESS ANALYSIS

A budget report has an internal purpose and an external purpose. The internal purpose of a budget report aids in making appropriate choices regarding operations. The external purpose of a budget report allows assessment of the feasibility and accountability of the program. A cost analysis includes accumulation, examination, and manipulation of cost data for comparisons and projections. A cost-effectiveness analysis is designed as a comparative tool to judge the relative costs and effects of courses of action to enable the selection of the action that will yield the most for the cost.

EMERGING TECHNOLOGY USEFUL TO HEALTH EDUCATION AND PROMOTION

BAM! (Body and Mind) is a website developed by the CDC for children ages 9 to 13 years old to help them to make good decisions about lifestyle choices. Children learn through games, quizzes, and interactive applications that use age-appropriate language. Activities for children include "Body-Image Ad Decoder" in which children measure dolls and action figures and compare measurements to normal body measurements. BAM! Provides support for educators through a number of activities and downloads as well as suggested lesson plans, which include evidence-based rationale for the activities.

65

While **pedometers** are less sophisticated than fitness trackers, they have many advantages such as being small, easy to use, and relatively inexpensive (starting at about $1). The user sets the normal stride and then turns on the pedometer, which monitors the number of footsteps and the distance covered. Some pedometers allow the data to be downloaded to a computer or other electronic device.

Diet and nutrition applications are available through app stores and websites for computers and mobile devices, such as smart phones and tablets. Some examples of free applications include DietHero, LoseIt!, Fooducate, Nutrino, and My Diet Coach. Diet and nutrition applications encourage people to diet and exercise, and some allow for groups of people to share information. While the applications vary somewhat, features that are fairly common include:

- Log for monitoring of weight
- Calculation of necessary calories for weight and height
- Calculation of calories burned for various activities and calories consumed
- Index of foods with calorie counts
- Recipes, food suggestions
- Tips for dealing with challenges, such as sugar cravings
- Barcode scanners for prepared foods
- Dieting diary
- Links to social media
- Rewards for personal challenges (drinking 8 glasses of water daily, parking at a distance)

Fitness trackers primarily track activity (such as steps taken) and calories burned, but some can also count the hours of sleep, the heart rate, and the skin temperature, making them useful for both fitness and cardiac monitoring. Fitness trackers range in price from less than $50 to hundreds of dollars. Some fit around the wrist (like a watch) while others clip on clothing. Issues to consider include:

- Type of display: Those that have a direct digital display (as opposed to those that simply send information to a computer or other device) provide immediate feedback.
- Waterproofing: Swimmers who want to track laps will need a fitness tracker that is waterproof.
- Battery life: Some must be recharged every 5 days while others run on 6-month watch batteries.
- Syncing ability: Some don't sync at all while others sync to computers, mobile devices, and even weight scales.
- Continuous or intermittent tracking: Some track 24 hours a day and others only during workout sessions.

Numerous smoking cessation applications are available through the app stores for computers and mobile devices, such as smartphones. **Smoking cessation applications** include a variety of different types:

- Financial calculators: These keep track of the dollar savings as people cut down their tobacco use or stop smoking altogether.
- Timers: These assist people to ration and decrease the frequency of their tobacco use by signaling according to a schedule set by the user.
- Self-hypnosis: These provide music or visualization exercises to help the person quit.

- Virtual reality: These allow people to smoke "virtual" cigarettes rather than succumbing to the desire for a real cigarette.
- Calendars: These tabulate the days without tobacco.

The National Cancer Institute has developed a free app, QuitPal, which combines many of the above features. Many more digital smoking cessation applications are under development.

OBTAINING PROGRAM SUPPORT

There are numerous communication strategies to obtain program support. One such strategy is that of social marketing. Social marketing is the use of marketing principles to promote a product, idea, or attitude. It involves setting behavioral goals, uses consumer research and theory, and targets populations. Health communication is an attempt to share information with, influence, and support a variety of audiences to engage in healthy behaviors or to support health-related policies, and is also vital. Numerous strategies may be employed in health communication. These strategies may include media, radio, TV, billboards, flyers, mail, email, and self-help literature.

When preparing a report to obtain or maintain support for a program, it is imperative to consider the audience for whom the report is prepared. The topic or purpose of the program should be clearly and concisely stated. A literature review with cited sources is needed to aid in defining the purpose of the study. Data must be explained and validated as well. It is important to present data in an understandable and clear way. Usually, a visual method such as the utilization of graphs or tables is the clearest form in which to present the data.

JUSTIFYING A PROGRAM

The type of **evidence** that would assist the health education specialist to justify a program varies according to the type of program but could include:

- Population data: A change in population, such as an increase in immigrants or older adults may indicate a need.
- Accreditation reports: Negative findings on accreditation review can be used to pinpoint needs and address the issues.
- Claims refusal data: High rates of claims refusals may indicate problems with care or coding.
- LOS and other census data: Because these directly relate to return-on-investment, if LOS exceeds that expected or census data shows decrease, then programs to counter this may be cost-effective.
- Infection/Sentinel event rates: High rates indicate a need for intervention because failing to intervene may increase liability.
- Needs assessment results: Indicates needs specific to the organization.
- Staffing shortages: Programs intended to retain staff or promote hiring may reduce shortages.
- Public health problems, trends: Public health data may indicate short-term or long-term needs.

COOPERATION AMONG STAKEHOLDERS

It is vital to facilitate cooperation among stakeholders responsible for health education. One should always demonstrate and maintain ethical behavior. It is imperative to have a firm understanding of the policies and the procedures of the institution. There also needs to be a dedicated understanding of the culture of the organization. Clear and effective communication with stakeholders will also facilitate cooperation. The communication with stakeholders may be intrapersonal, interpersonal, or formal. In order to facilitate cooperation among stakeholders, it is important that one exhibit and

67

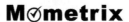

understand cultural competency. Finally, maintaining objectivity is a key element in facilitating cooperation.

FORMING A COALITION

Health educators will often form a coalition when implementing a health education program. In the field, a coalition is defined as a group of people working towards the same goal. These people may represent disparate organizations and have different areas of expertise, but they are all focused on solving the same problem. One of the benefits of forming a coalition is that it allows a health educator to get fresh perspectives from a number of different points of view. Individuals with different professional backgrounds are likely to approach the same problem from different angles, and a health educator overseeing the program can pick and choose the ideas that he or she prefers.

EVALUATING THE FEASIBILITY OF CONTINUING PARTNERSHIP

Effective partnerships require continued preparation, planning, implementation, evaluation, and sustainability. To evaluate the feasibility of continuing a partnership, the following must be assessed: mutual benefit (to include public health enhancement), improvement in outreach, decreased duplication of services, broadened base of support, improved credibility, and increased appeal to those funding the program. It is also important to ensure that trust has been established, end goals have been determined, accountability is shared, and that "turf battles" have been minimized. It is also crucial to compare the results of the program to resources saved or utilized and to reevaluate the goals and the missions of the partnership.

SYNTHESIZING DATA FOR REPORTING

It is important to use meta-analysis when synthesizing data for the purposes of reporting. Meta-analysis refers to combining results to answer research hypotheses. Meta-analysis is a vital component of a systematic review process of the data obtained. There are numerous advantages to using meta-analysis. Such advantages include the ability to tell if the results are more varied than what is expected from the sample diversity, derivation and statistical testing of overall factors/effect size parameters in related studies, generalization to the population of studies, ability to control for between-study variation, and the use of moderators to explain variation.

META-ANALYSIS

There are several approaches to meta-analysis. One such approach is that of vote-counting. Vote-counting defines findings as significantly positive (in favor of the treatment group), significantly negative, or non-significant. The finding with the most is thought to be the one that best represents the research; vote-counting is considered to be an inexact means of data synthesis. Another approach is that of classic or Glassian meta-analysis. Classic meta-analysis defines questions to be examined, collects studies, codes study features and outcomes, and analyzes relations between study features and outcomes.

LEARNING LEADERSHIP SKILLS

Insofar as they are charged with administering a health education program, a health educator will have to function effectively as a leader. This means setting a good example for cooperation, responsibility, and diligence. It also means establishing a clear chain of command and channels of communication for staff. A continuous flow of information throughout an organization makes it possible for all members of staff to make appropriate decisions. An organizational leader is also responsible for setting appropriate priorities and making sure that all efforts are aimed at achieving the most important objectives.

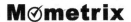

ORGANIZATIONAL LEADERSHIP

A health educator will have to exhibit some organizational leadership skills in order to manage his or her program. The role of the organizational leader is to set up administrative structures that allow the goals of the organization to be realized. One of the most important ways that an organizational leader will affect the health of the program is by establishing channels of communication. It is essential that there is an uninhibited flow of information throughout the organization so that inefficiencies can be avoided. An organizational leader also needs to make sure that there is a clear chain of command in the organization, so that there will not be any questions regarding authority or responsibility.

ORGANIZATIONAL CULTURE

The culture of an organization is the set of beliefs and behaviors that it deems acceptable and appropriate. The general parameters of organizational culture are established by the mission statement and goals of the program: accepted beliefs and practices will be those that contribute to the accomplishment of goals. Organizational culture will also be established by strong leaders who represent the core values they wish to see promoted in the program. A strong organizational culture gives a program a kind of forward momentum and has a self-reinforcing effect on the work of the program. If the culture of the organization is supportive, staff members will feel comfortable bringing any concerns they might have to management.

In order to facilitate change within organizational cultures, it is important to assess the culture and its capacity for change. The following are some strategies to use: innovative ideas and taking risks, careful attention to detail, outcome-orientation, population-orientation, team-orientation, aggressiveness, and stability. A certified health education specialist may also facilitate organizational change by giving technical assistance, being an advocate, engaging in strategic planning, building and providing support for teams, and facilitating and implementing various interventions. It is also important to be actively involved in management building and structural redesign.

SYSTEMS APPROACH TO CHANGE

The systems approach to change is thought to be the best method by which to approach organizational change. The systems approach entails breaking the project down into parts that are connected in a logical manner, and studying/analyzing the parts of the project in order to ascertain how these parts perform. Organizational change is vital to health education because such change facilitates the development of new programs of health education and the implementation of new programs within organizations. Organizational change is necessary for the adoption and implementation of new policies.

STRATEGIC PLANNING

Strategic planning is the laying out of long-term goals and the tasks it will take to accomplish them. In order to be comprehensive, strategic planning must include reference to all aspects of the program. As much as possible, individuals engaged in strategic planning should try to consider possible obstacles to success, and how these obstacles may be overcome. It is certain that strategic plans will need to be occasionally revised as problems and inefficiencies emerge.

There are three important concerns that a health educator should keep in mind while developing long-term strategic plans. To begin with, a health educator needs to make sure that he or she has an accurate perception of the current situation. It will be impossible to set reasonable goals and estimate potential resources without first achieving an accurate appreciation of the organization as it stands. Second, a health educator needs to set goals to organize the planning efforts. All

69

objectives should be designed in order to reach the agreed-upon long-term goals. The effort to create tasks that lead directly to the accomplishment of these objectives is the third major concern of a health educator during the planning period.

A health educator should follow a step-by-step protocol in developing long-term plans for his or her program:

- Organize a planning committee
- Set basic organizational goals
- Identify stakeholders and determine how best to advance their interests
- Perform a comprehensive resource inventory
- Set priorities for administrative action
- Plan strategies for addressing the core needs of the program
- Confer with stakeholders regarding the suitability of the plans
- Set a timeline for the accomplishment of tasks, objectives, and goals
- Implement the program and make any necessary changes to the program plan

PROMOTING COOPERATION AND FEEDBACK AMONG PROGRAM-RELATED PERSONNEL

When the culture of an organization is positive and supportive, the staff will feel comfortable working together and giving their honest judgments on program-related subjects. This is essential because in any program, individuals will have varying areas of interest and levels of expertise, and a leader will need to hear honest reports from all members of staff. Organizational leaders need to get as much feedback as possible from members of staff, so that they can make informed decisions regarding the continuation of program components. The leader of a program should take care to encourage staff members to provide feedback whenever appropriate.

APPLICATION OF HUMAN RESOURCE POLICIES

There are many ways in which to manage human resources in an effective manner that will comply with relevant laws and regulations. It is important to understand leadership methods that involve participation and also to consider various work style diversity. One should also acknowledge and respect the abilities and the talents of the members of the group as well as utilize the strengths of the members of the group to attain the objectives and the goals of the program and its mission. There are numerous federal laws and regulations to be considered.

FEDERAL LAWS

LAWS PROHIBITING EMPLOYEE DISCRIMINATION AND PROTECTING EMPLOYMENT RIGHTS

The federal laws that prohibit employee discrimination are as follows: Title VII of the Civil Rights Act, Civil Rights Act of 1991, Age Discrimination in Employment Act, Americans with Disabilities Act of 1990, Rehabilitation Act of 1973, Pregnancy Discrimination Act of 1978, Vietnam Veterans Readjustment Assistance Act of 1974, Fair Credit Reporting and Disclosure Act, and the Immigration Reform and Control Act of 1986. The federal laws that protect employment rights are as follows: Family Medical Leave Act of 1993 and the Worker's Compensation Act. There are also federal laws that protect employee benefits and compensation.

LAWS THAT PROTECT EMPLOYEE BENEFITS AND THAT APPLY TO HUMAN RESOURCES

The federal laws that protect employee benefits and compensation are as follows: the Fair Labor Standards Act, the Employee Retirement Income Security Act of 1974, the Consolidated Omnibus Budget Reconciliation Act (COBRA), and the Unemployment Compensation Equal Pay Act of 1963. There are several other federal laws that apply to human resources. These laws are as follows: the

National Labor Relations Act of 1935, Worker Adjustment and Retraining Notification Act of 1988, the Occupational Safety and Health Act of 1970 (OSHA), and the Health Insurance Portability and Accountability Act of 1996 (HIPAA).

ULTIMATE RESPONSIBILITY

According to the Code of Ethics, the ultimate responsibility of a health educator is to provide information for the promotion and maintenance of health. This can be done at the individual, family, or community level. At all times, however, a health educator needs to respect the autonomy and freedom of choice of those individuals with whom they work. Indeed, the foundations of ethical professional practice are promoting good, promoting social justice, avoiding harm, and respecting the autonomy of the individual.

DEVELOPING VOLUNTEER OPPORTUNITIES

Many health programs rely on the contributions of volunteers for much of the important organizational work. Large programs will often recruit volunteers in advertisements and public service announcements. Although volunteers are a blessing for a health program, they do need to be interviewed and trained before they are allowed to begin work. Volunteers cannot be expected to be aware of every aspect of an operational health program, so they must be closely monitored to ensure that they stay on track. At all times, volunteers should be treated with respect and warmth.

ENHANCING STAFF MEMBERS' AND VOLUNTEERS' CAREER DEVELOPMENT

There are four key elemental tasks when working with volunteers. It is important to recruit, train, supervise, and recognize. Volunteers need evaluations or performance reviews just as staff members need evaluations and performance reviews. It is critical to utilize team building activities when working with staff members and with volunteers. Team-building activities include the setting of goals, the development of interpersonal relationships, clarification of roles and responsibilities, and careful process analysis. It is also important to provide career training for both staff members and volunteers. Such training may be used in new employee orientation as well.

CAREER TRAINING AND EMPLOYEE APPRAISALS

Career training is an essential part of enhancing staff members' and volunteers' career development. Such training improves the performances of staff members and volunteers. It also serves to update technology skills and to provide information on changes within the organization or changes in management. Career training will also help to provide solutions to problems in the organization and help to prepare an employee for promotion within the organization. Employee appraisals are helpful and serve to aid the leadership of the organization. Appraisals provide information to help with administrative decisions, performance information, information regarding the skills of employees and of supervisors, and information regarding the ability of management to change employees' performances.

PERFORMANCE EVALUATIONS OF STAFF AND VOLUNTEERS

Performance evaluations of both staff and volunteers are important tools in the success of a program or a project. Such evaluations will provide information for managers, administrators, and individuals. Such evaluations aid in identifying strengths and weaknesses, in providing improved accountability for resource utilization, and in improving morale. Performance evaluations should include the performance of the individual staff member or volunteer, the efficiency of the program, and the effectiveness of the program. A performance evaluation should include a self-evaluation of the staff member or volunteer as well as an external evaluation by managers.

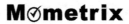

CONFLICT RESOLUTION

Conflict resolution directs individuals and organizations to see similarities and differences that exist between them and then leads them to focus on reducing differences in order to accomplish goals and objectives. The steps in conflict resolution are to create an atmosphere for goal accomplishment; clarify perceptions of those involved; focus on needs of individuals and organizations as separate entities as well as the needs of collective individuals and organizations; build shared positive power; work toward a future orientation; create options; develop goals, objectives, and activities that can be accomplished; and make sure that all involved benefit.

There are many effective conflict resolution strategies. It is important to be well-prepared by looking at one's own behavior first. It is essential to take responsibility for one's own part in the conflict and to openly discuss the effect of the conflict. Conflict needs to be resolved in a timely fashion since it becomes more difficult to resolve if allowed to build and fester. Discussions regarding conflict need to occur in a private and neutral area. Physical barriers to positive communication need to be removed. The problem needs to be clearly identified, and one must listen in an active manner.

Serve as a Health Education/Promotion Resource Person

HUMAN CLEARINGHOUSE

A clearinghouse is an institution charged with assembling and distributing information. A health educator is often referred to as a "human clearinghouse" because he or she has to collect information and make sure it is distributed to all pertinent members of staff. There are a number of different sources for information on health and education. Some of the most important sources will pertain to the community in which the program is placed. More general information can be found in the Educational Resources Information Center or the National Health Information Clearinghouse databases.

ASSESSMENT OF INFORMATION NEEDS

When serving as a health education resource person, it is important to assess information needs. The information needs of a population first have to be defined. There are several methods by which to define the information needs of a population. One method is to obtain statistics for community assessment or formative research. Educational materials are also used to define the need for information. Another method is to use evidence-based programs or strategies for program planning. Survey tools or evaluations for data collection may also be useful in defining the information needs of a population. Finally, topic-specific information may also serve as a tool in assessing information needs.

BEING ASKED TO PROVIDE HEALTH INFORMATION

FIVE-STEP PROCESS A TO FOLLOW WHEN ASKED TO PROVIDE HEALTH INFORMATION

When health educators are asked to provide health information, there is a specific five step process that they should follow. This protocol has been established to organize the efforts of health professionals in this regard. The first step is to honestly assess the needs of the target community. This can be done by analyzing data or by conducting interviews. The health professional should then determine which information sources will directly meet the needs of the target community. The health professional can then access these resources. At this point, he or she will want to look over the materials and assess their reliability, validity, and quantity. Finally, before presenting the information to the client, the health professionals should organize the material in an easy-to-understand format.

FINDING VALID SOURCES OF INFORMATION TO PROVIDE

It is very common for a health educator to be asked to provide information on a subject out of their range of expertise. For this reason, health educators need to be able to refer people to the right sources for reliable and accurate information. Also, a health educator needs to be able to find information that is at the right level of sophistication for the interested party. Some of the resources that a health educator might turn to are the Internet, government literature, or pamphlets from nongovernmental agencies. When providing information to a curious individual, a health educator needs to take care that the information is reliable and recent.

SOURCES OF OBTAINING INFORMATION

In order to stay abreast of the most current information in health education, a health educator has to be familiar with the most important sources of health knowledge. The two most common

73

professional databases used by health educators are administered by the National Health Information Clearinghouse and the Educational Resources Information Center. These databases contain all the latest journal articles and government reports concerning health education. There are some other databases that contain education articles, including the International Health Education E-Mail Directory and the Combined Health Information Database.

COMPUTER-RELATED INFORMATION

There are a number of different venues for obtaining health information:

- Internet: Health-related websites, health-themed search engines
- Health CD-ROMs
- Professional journals: Most of these maintain online archives
- Online databases: ERIC, MEDLINE, PsychLIT, etc.

DATABASES AND DATA ANALYSIS SYSTEMS

There are a number of databases and data analysis systems available to health educators:

- HealthFinder: A website maintained by the US government
- Spreadsheets: Used to organize and perform calculations on large sets of numerical data
- Statistical Analysis software: used to determine data trends
- Health-risk appraisal software: Used to calculate the likelihood of adverse health consequences for various individuals in various circumstances

PRIMARY, SECONDARY, AND TERTIARY SOURCES OF HEALTH INFORMATION

Health educators distinguish primary, secondary, and tertiary sources of health information.

- Primary sources: All the objective, numerical research data published in journal articles, databases, and other professional literature
- Secondary sources: Assemblages of data taken indirectly, as for instance from journal articles that compile a number of different research studies
- Tertiary sources: Collections of data taken from both primary and secondary sources; commonly found in government publications and organizational summaries

ONLINE SOURCES OF INFORMATION FOR HEALTH EDUCATORS

MEDLINE is the database assembled by the United States National Library of Medicine. This database has a focus on biomedicine, but also contains scholarly articles on public health and medical research. Although entries in the database are predominantly from scholarly journals, there are also newspaper articles, magazine columns, and newsletters. Most of the articles on this site can be accessed for free, though others require a small fee. There is no fee charged for search privileges. Search results will include a brief abstract of each article.

> MEDLINE: (http://ncbi.nlm.nih.gov/PubMed) Database maintained by the United States National Library of Medicine; includes references to health education journals and medical journals

The Education Resources Information Center, known as ERIC, is a comprehensive education database organized by the Institute of Education Sciences administered by the United States Department of Education. This database focuses on scholarly articles related to K-12 education. At present, ERIC contains upwards of one million articles, and in time will include audio and video files. For the most part, materials can be accessed for no charge. ERIC contains materials from all over the world.

> ERIC: (http://www.eric.ed.gov/) Database of education journals, with an emphasis on K-12 education

The Combined Health Information Database, known as CHID, is administered by the National Institute of health. This database contains articles about health education programs in the following fields: Alzheimer's disease; complementary and alternative medicine; deafness and communication disorders; diabetes; digestive diseases; kidney and urologic diseases; maternal and child health; medical genetics and rare disorders; oral health; and weight control. The intent of CHID is to provide access to instructional materials and research articles that cannot be found elsewhere.

> CHID: (http://www.chid.nih.gov) Includes information about current health education programs; includes article titles and abstracts

Health educators frequently find themselves consulting the Combined Health Information Database to discover more information about a particular topic. The 10 topics covered in depth by this database are among the most frequent sources of professional inquiry by health educators. For school educators, as an example, the section on weight control will be particularly useful when developing nutrition and fitness plans for students. Many health educators these days find themselves working in consultation with school districts to develop healthy meals and alternatives to junk food in public schools.

The Cumulative Index for Nursing and Allied Health Literature, known by the acronym CINAHL, is a collection of nursing articles and other resources for medical professionals. This database provides access to books, journal articles, dissertations, and conference meetings on a variety of subjects related to nursing and Allied health. In addition, members of this database receive access to MEDLINE. Individuals may purchase year long memberships to CINAHL.

> CINAHL: (http://www.cinahl.com/) Lists the articles in health education journals

Health and Psychosocial Instruments, known by the abbreviation HaPI, is a collection of information regarding data collection tools. HaPI houses thousands of surveys, scales, tests, and rating schemes that have been used in previous research experiments. These data collection instruments are predominantly geared towards measuring pain, quality of life, and drug efficacy. The tests are drawn from the following fields of research: medical, social, physical therapy, psychology, and speech and hearing therapy.

> HaPI: (http://www.ovid.com) contains information about reliable and valid methods for evaluating health programs

HEDIR AND HEALTHPROM

HEDIR, the international electronic mail directory for health educators, is a great way to contact knowledgeable professionals all over the world. Health educators who register with the directory gain access to the professional expertise of colleagues in every conceivable field of health education. HEALTHPROM is another email directory of health educators; its name is short for "health promotion." HEALTHPROM emphasizes the health concerns of mothers, newborns, and children in Eastern Europe and Central Asia.

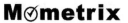

Role of Governmental and Nongovernmental Agencies in Providing Health Information

Health educators will often need to rely on both governmental and nongovernmental agencies to provide health information. Some of the most well-known nongovernmental agencies that provide a wealth of health information are the American Cancer Society, the Red Cross, and the American Heart Association. All of these groups are excellent resources for specific health information. Governmental agencies like the CDC and the NIH are also fabulous repositories of health data. These institutions make their research findings available to health professionals as a free resource.

Scenario One

You are a health educator hired to help plan a dental hygiene program in an elementary school.

Identify some of the resources you might utilize to obtain information.

A health educator who's been hired to plan a dental hygiene program in an elementary school might begin by interviewing some of the local experts. These might include school health officials and dentists. It's important to identify which dental hygiene issues are most pertinent for the target population of students. Journal articles can also be a useful source of ideas. Finally, the health educator might want to consult some of the professional organizations, as for instance the American School Health Association or the Directors of Health Promotion and Education.

Gathering Resource Information

There are a number of ways for health educators to gather resource information. Government agencies publish extensive reports of the research they are commissioned to perform, and they often create multimedia presentation formats for health educators. Nongovernmental agencies also are good sources of resource information, as they are in part funded to promote health issues through the dissemination of literature and individual presentations. Many school and university libraries will maintain an extensive collection of health-related resources that can be checked out and used.

Accessing Educational Resources That Will Aid Individuals and Community Groups

In order to provide the most helpful educational resources to the members of the target community, health educators need to be familiar with the most common points of access. These days, the best way to get in touch with the purveyors of health information is through the Internet. Health educators should be familiar with the websites of all major nongovernmental agencies as well as those departments of the federal government that offer education resources. Another frequently used website is the Gateway to Educational Materials, which provides a wealth of health-related lesson plans and presentation guides.

Responding When Asked to Provide Health Information

Health educators are constantly being asked to lend their expertise to health issues in public and private settings. Part of being an effective educator is knowing which resources are appropriate for which situation. For instance, sophisticated clients should be given access to the scholarly articles that a trained health educator reviews. Less educated clients, on the other hand, may be given materials that are easier to understand. When serving as a consultant, a health educator needs to work in close communication with the client in order to ascertain which materials are appropriate.

AVAILABLE INFORMATION SOURCES FOR THE HEALTH EDUCATOR

There are numerous available information sources for the health educator. Such sources include: United States Census, National Center for Health Statistics, Government Printing Office website, Medline Plus, Health finder, Health on the Net, Gateway to Educational Materials (GEM), Health Resources and Services Administration (HRSA), National Health Information Center, ERIC database, CHID database, CINAHL database, EBMR database, HaPl database, PsychInfo database. There are also evidence-based strategies on the internet. Such strategies include National Cancer Institute's Research-Tested Interventions, Diffusion of Effective Behavioral Interventions for HIV Programs, SAMSHA's Guide to Evidence-based Practices, and the National Registry of Evidence-Based Programs and Practices.

ASSESSING INFORMATION FOUND ONLINE

USING A COMPUTER TO DETERMINE THE RELEVANCE OF HEALTH INFORMATION

It can be difficult to wade through the huge amount of health literature on the Internet. In order to be efficient and provide only the most high-quality data, educators need to become adept at sorting through a high volume of sources. The best way to do this is to quickly assess the reliability of a website by examining its documentation, references, and credentials. Also, educators should try to use the most recent research findings whenever possible.

QUESTIONS TO USE WHEN ASSESSING INFORMATION

There are a few basic considerations that can be made when determining whether to trust the information from a certain website. To begin with, one can examine the operator of the site. Is it a licensed and well-known organization? A reliable website will declare its credentials and will include links to other well-known health websites. These other websites are intended to function as a sort of "second opinion," confirming the assertions of the original website. It is also a good idea to check out the credentials of the authors of the content you are using. Have they received degrees or citations from noteworthy institutions? The most reliable websites on the Internet will be only too glad to demonstrate their authority.

Health educators are frequently required to seek out new information on health-related topics. The Internet is increasingly a site of research and commentary on these issues. However, the free and open nature of the Internet means that health educators must be conscious of only taking information from reputable sources. Websites that are maintained by government agencies, universities, and nonprofit groups can be assumed to be as accurate as possible. Websites that display a list of editors, and include the credentials of these editors, can also be trusted. It is likewise encouraging when websites display a list of links to well-established websites, which serve as a sort of "second opinion." Finally, websites that are frequently updated are more likely to be maintained by individuals or groups with a strong commitment to delivering accurate health information.

CRITERIA TO USE WHEN EVALUATING A WEBSITE AND THE INFORMATION IT CONTAINS

There is so much information related to health on the Internet these days, it can be overwhelming to an educator. Unfortunately, much of this material is not adequately researched or evaluated by experts. When examining a website, therefore, a health educator needs to determine whether an editorial board has reviewed the information. The best websites will include the credentials of those individuals who have performed editorial duties. Another mark of quality in a health-related website is a set of links to other, similar websites. Quality websites will be frequently updated in accordance with new research findings. In general, you can tell a great deal about the quality of a website by its condition. Government websites tend to be well maintained and frequently updated, and they are among the most reputable sources of health information on the Internet.

SCENARIO TWO

You are a health educator contracted to work with a personal care home whose residents have Alzheimer's disease.

Using four key questions, determine the credibility of information gathered from the following websites:

1. A blog entry dated 3/7/14 from a website called vitaminsdiary.com. It cites a study at Tufts University showing that blueberries may help ward off Alzheimer's. No links are provided.
2. A newsletter from ADEAR, the Alzheimer's & related Dementias Education & Referral Center (alzheimers.gov)
3. A list of articles concerning Alzheimer's on MedlinePlus.

As always, when dealing with information found on the Internet it is important to pay attention to the source. In general, the information found on websites like ADEAR and MedlinePlus will be more reliable and accurate than that found on a blog like vitaminsdiary.com. For one thing, the blog entry in question is a couple of years old. It also does not refer to its sources, so there is no way to confirm the veracity of the account. Websites like ADEAR and MedlinePlus are careful to provide references and contact information. For this reason, their claims can be taken more seriously.

ENSURING THAT INFORMATION GATHERED AND PRESENTED WILL BE USEFUL

Health educators are constantly working to promote their programs among the members of the target population. In order to be effective in this role, the health educator needs to make sure that the information presented to the public is easy to understand and accurate. Information should also be presented in an organized fashion. It is counterproductive to disseminate information that contains a great deal of unfamiliar vocabulary and complicated health concepts. Also, a health educator should take care not to overwhelm the target population with a high volume of information.

There are a few general considerations that a health educator must keep in mind in order to ensure that the information gathered and presented in a program will be useful to the target audience:

- Material must engage the audience, meaning that the audience is attentive and interested.
- All information must be accurate and up to date.
- Information must be presented in an easy-to-understand, orderly manner.
- Information should not reach a level of detail inappropriate to the understanding of the audience.
- As much as possible, information should be applicable to the lives of the audience.
- Vocabulary should neither too sophisticated nor too simplistic for the target audience.
- Clear and appropriate graphics should accompany the presentation.

APPROPRIATE VOCABULARY AND MATERIAL

As any health educator knows, the literature on a given subject will range from extremely simple to extraordinarily complex. Although a health educator may be trained to understand even the most sophisticated writing on a health subject, he or she must keep in mind that the members of the target population most likely are not. For this reason, it is important that all information that disseminated to the target population is free of unfamiliar jargon and scientific or medical terminology. Some members of the target community will be alienated by unfamiliar language and may decide for this reason not to participate in the health program.

SCENARIO THREE

You are a health educator under contract to a retirement home. You have implemented a program to promote heart health, but the residents complain that printed materials are filled with "newfangled words" such as "thromboembolism" and "anticoagulants".

Explain what steps you would take to minimize those complaints.

It is your job as a health educator to make sure the target population is able to understand the information you provide. If senior citizens are complaining that the language in your pamphlets and brochures is too technical, you have a couple of different options. First, you could try to explain the definitions above those words which are unavoidable and essential to understanding of the health issue. You could also provide some new materials that use more colloquial language. Sometimes, you might be able to explain the meanings of esoteric words by incorporating illustrations and charts.

SCENARIO FOUR

You are a health educator working for a company which manufactures automobiles. You have developed a large packet of materials to help workers prevent injuries caused by repetitive motion, but many workers admit they have not really looked at the material because "there's too much reading."

Explain what steps you would take to minimize those complaints.

Obviously, the quality of your written information will be irrelevant if you cannot persuade the target population to read it. In this case, it seems that it will be necessary to provide information in a more "easy to digest" format. One way to do this would be to provide materials with more illustrations and visual representations. You will also probably need to condense the written information. It is important to isolate the most important information, especially those pieces of practical advice that employees will be able to use to help resolve the health problem.

SCENARIO FIVE

You are a health educator planning a dental hygiene program for high school students in an inner-city school.

Explain why a brochure featuring "Timmy the Talking Tooth" would not be an appropriate material. Also, provide a suggestion for material that would be appropriate.

When you are distributing information on a health related subject, you need to make sure that the sophistication of your material is appropriate for the target population. High school students are probably too old and cynical to accept the advice of "Timmy the Talking Tooth." Indeed, high school students would probably stop listening to a presentation that they feel is far below their level of intellectual sophistication. It would be more appropriate to give the students some pamphlets or brochures that contain statistics and basic information on dental hygiene. High school students are also old enough to see some graphic depictions of decayed teeth and gums.

REQUESTS FOR TRAINING

When presented with requests for training, it is essential to carefully investigate the request to ascertain whether the request will be a good fit with the needs of the organization. The request for training should also be analyzed to assure that such a request will yield positive outcomes for the participants. It is necessary to identify the priority populations who will receive the most benefit from training and to identify who has a lack of knowledge or of skills. The primary stakeholders also need to be identified, and the time, budget, and personnel needed for training also need to be addressed.

PRIORITIZING TRAINING REQUESTS

When attempting to prioritize requests for training, it is necessary to consider many aspects. One of the aspects to consider is the urgency of the need for training. The objectives of the training need to be considered as well. Another aspect to think about is the potential impact of the training. Another factor to consider would be the range of impact of the training. The training design and the needs of such a design will also require investigation. The size of the audience is an important factor. The requestor as well as the costs and the anticipated workload are also aspects to consider.

TRAINING NEEDS ASSESSMENT

There are numerous areas to be considered and addressed when conducting a training needs assessment. Initially, the training need should be identified. The design of the needs assessment will need to be ascertained. The collection of pertinent data is required. Analysis of the collected data is also a necessity. Feedback is an important area of assessment of training needs. The following are examples of possible questions to assess training needs: What type of training have you had in order to prepare you for your job? What are the most difficult parts of your job? What additional training do you need in order to perform your job better?

IDENTIFICATION OF EXISTING RESOURCES THAT MEET TRAINING NEEDS

When preparing to meet training needs, it is essential to identify existing resources that meet such needs. The following questions regarding existing resources should be addressed: Does the resource contain the information that the client/community wants to know? Can the client/community understand the information contained in the resource? Is the information current and accurate? Is the format appropriate and the information culturally appropriate? Will the resource meet the program objectives? What is the reading level of the materials? A good existing resource is the Gateway to Educational Materials (GEM), which provides numerous educational resources.

DEVELOPMENT OF A TRAINING PLAN

There are numerous elements to be considered when developing an effective training plan. The training needs must be identified and the objectives determined. The content of the subject to fulfill the objectives needs to be decided. The participants in the training need to be chosen. A training schedule will need to be established. A facility in which to provide the training must be obtained. Instructors for the training need to be contacted and hired. Audiovisual aids need to be chosen and prepared. The program needs to be coordinated. Finally, the program will need to be evaluated.

FACILITATING COLLABORATIVE TRAINING EFFORTS WITH DIFFERENT ORGANIZATIONS

Sometimes, a health educator will find that it is essential to provide collaborative training to individuals from different organizations. For instance, a health educator might determine that in order for the employees of local health-care facilities to provide adequate and appropriate services to the target population it is necessary for them to be educated on the subject of the health education program. In order for the training to be effective, health educators should limit its content to what is essential for each party participating. Also, one of the goals of the training should be to improve the relationships between the constituent organizations.

IMPLEMENTATION OF A TRAINING PLAN

After forming a training plan, a training implementation plan will need to be instituted. The training plan implementation should include an explanation of the administrative details. The training implementation plan also will need details on the means by which the training will be promoted. Information about the recruitment of the target audience is a necessary aspect of the training implementation plan. The training objectives will need to be described carefully as well. The mechanism for the evaluation of the training also needs to be illustrated and the budget carefully set forth.

TEACHING STRATEGIES AND TRAINING EVALUATION

There are multiple teaching strategies that may be used in training. The use of lectures and case studies is a useful teaching strategy. Discussion and demonstration are two effective strategies that may be used in training. The use of peer groups is another means of teaching. Audiovisual and print aids and materials can be utilized as training devices. Multimedia and simulations may also be employed as training strategies. Training will need to be evaluated in order to ensure that it is useful and should be continued, and to collect information for improvement.

TRAINING LEVELS THAT NEED TO BE EVALUATED

The levels of training that need to evaluated include reaction (level 1), learning (level 2), behavior (level 3), and results (level 4). The description of and the tools necessary for level 1 (reaction) are the feelings of the participants regarding the training and involve using surveys and feedback forms. Level 2 (learning) includes the extent of attitude change, knowledge gained, or increase in skills, and uses a pre- and post-survey. Level 3 is described as the extent to which the participants are using job skills; tools include interviews and observations. Level 4 is described as the organizational effects; tools include document review for success indicators.

CONSULTATION

Health educators are occasionally required to serve as consultants in order to provide access to the appropriate materials and resources to solve a particular health problem. Sometimes, businesses or other organizations decide that they want to address a particular health problem, but they have no employees with any expertise. If the business does not want to hire a full-time health professional, it may elect to hire a health educator as a consultant for a limited period of time. When the health educator assigns a written contract, this is known as formal consulting. The extent to which the health educator participates in the planning, implementation, and evaluation of the health program is determined by the client.

> **Review Video: Steps in Consultation**
> Visit mometrix.com/academy and enter code: 566019

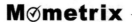

INFORMAL CONSULTING VS. FORMAL CONSULTING

Health educators are often asked to lend their professional expertise to a health-related problem in another setting. For instance, businesses may consult with a health educator when they are faced with health problems. Sometimes, the health educator's role as a consultant is informal, meaning that the educator simply gathers and organizes appropriate professional materials. At other times, however, a health educator will sign a contract with the client, and will perform consulting services on a formal basis. In these cases, the health educator will take a much more involved approach to recommending and assisting with the implementation of health solutions.

INTERNAL CONSULTING VS. EXTERNAL CONSULTING

Because of their expertise on health-related issues, health educators are often called upon to act as consultants for schools and businesses. In this role, the health educator needs to make sure that he or she is functioning within the parameters of the position as specified by the client organization. One of the most important functions that a health educator performs as a consultant is as a clearinghouse for health information; often times, schools and businesses simply do not know where to look to find the appropriate information. By connecting individuals and organizations with accurate and reliable health information, educators promote positive changes in behavior.

Consulting is considered to be external when the health educator is providing information or guidance to an organization that they normally do not work with. In order for this consulting relationship to be effective, it is typical for a contract to be drawn up outlining the responsibilities and duties of the health educator. In a usual external consulting task, the health educator will organize all the health-related information pertinent to the topic of interest to the organization and then develop a program to resolve whatever problems exist. Basically, organizations will hire an external consultant to deal with a health problem which they do not understand.

PRIORITIZING CONSULTANT REQUESTS

When serving as a health education consultant, it is important to prioritize requests for assistance. The request must be in congruence with the skills of the consultant. The area in which the request falls with regard to the services that are offered will also need to be considered. The scope and nature of the request for consultation must also be addressed. The level of commitment required of the request is another element for consideration. It is also necessary to determine if other consultants may be available who could provide services.

ESTABLISHING AND CONTINUING CONSULTING USING NETWORKING

Health educators constantly are making connections with consumer groups, local leaders, and health care experts. These connections can be a wonderful resource. Indeed, many health educators are offered consulting positions based on their long relationship with an organization. Organizations will be more likely to offer a consulting position to a health educator with whom they are familiar and whom they believe has a strong knowledge of their operations. Furthermore, health educators will be much more able to immediately assist an organization with which he or she is familiar. By building close working relationships in the community, a health educator can advance his or her own career while providing superior service.

APPLYING ETHICAL PRINCIPLES FOR EFFECTIVE CONSULTATIVE RELATIONSHIPS

The consultative relationship is kept more effective and more ethical with monitoring of the progress and the facilitation of open communication. It is vital to utilize continuous evaluation in a consultative relationship and also for the CHES not to officially serve as an advocate for the client while involved in a consultative relationship. The CHES should use the following steps for a consultative evaluation: identification of evaluation questions and criteria, assessment of how well

82

the questions meet the criteria, and timely distribution of the findings. The following criteria are used for the consultant's formative evaluation: number and length of contacts, progress made, and level of client satisfaction.

HEALTH EDUCATOR AS LIAISON

BETWEEN STAFF AND OUTSIDE ORGANIZATIONS

Sometimes, it will be necessary for a health educator to act as a liaison between departments in the same organization or in two different organizations. This underscores the importance of open channels for communication when dealing with health issues. As the departments or organizations struggle to resolve a health issue, the health educator will make sure that each side is apprised of progress and actions being taken by the other. Also, the health educator will be available to answer questions as they arise. In this role, the health educator needs to focus on making each constituent department or organization as efficient as possible.

BETWEEN CONSUMER GROUPS, INDIVIDUALS, AND HEALTH CARE PROVIDERS

Occasionally, a health educator will be called upon to serve as a liaison between consumer groups, individuals, and health care providers. For instance, a health educator may need to work with health care providers to ensure that the individuals in the target community are receiving appropriate care that reinforces the objectives of the health education program. At other times, a health educator may partner with local consumer groups to promote changes in policy that will advance health objectives. By maintaining relationships with all three of these groups, and by facilitating communication among them, health educators can establish a positive attitude towards their program in the community.

EXPERTISE NEEDED

The certified health education specialist may provide a great deal of expertise in a consultative relationship. One area of expertise is that of health education and health promotion. The CHES also has the skills for program assessment, program planning, and program evaluation. A CHES consultant is a good resource for health education resources and health education materials. The CHES consultant may also contribute professional guidance regarding health-related procedures. The consultant can be utilized as a liaison between individuals, between groups, and between health care provider organizations. A liaison will require the following skills: facilitation, presentation, data collection, meeting management, resource evaluation, networking, and report writing.

ACTING AS RESOURCES IN DIFFERENT SETTINGS

Health educators will serve as resources in a variety of different settings. In schools, they will need to provide information to school administrators and policymakers so that appropriate health-related decisions can be made. They will also have to provide information to students. When employed by a healthcare facility, they will have to disseminate information to patients and staff alike. When working in a business, they will have to provide health information to management regarding the efficacy of health education programs, and to employees regarding the benefits of positive health-related changes.

SOURCE OF INFORMATION TERMS

- Consultation: the health educator gives advice to another person so that the other person can make a good decision
- Informal consulting: a health educator helps a professional partner by assembling information and analyzing data; no written agreement required
- Formal consulting: health educator uses his or her professional expertise to recommend solutions to a health problem; involves a written agreement between educator and client

Communicate, Promote, and Advocate for Health

HEALTH EDUCATORS AND COMMUNICATION

Health educators have a responsibility to disseminate information that is reliable, accurate, and current. They also are responsible for presenting information in such a way that it can be readily understood by those individuals it affects. A health educator, in order to make a positive difference, needs to have an accurate understanding of his or her audience. At times, it may be necessary for a health educator to prioritize his or her objectives and to communicate only the information that will lead to the accomplishment of the most important objectives.

The following are key terms related to health education communication and advocacy:

- Culture: the set of values and behavior patterns that is common to a group, whether explicitly or tacitly
- Advocacy: efforts to call attention to a health issue
- Persuasive communication: efforts to encourage a target population to make positive behavior changes by providing information and advice
- Health communication: the dissemination of health-related information in a target community
- Health marketing: the use of commercial marketing principles to promote health behavior

HEALTH COMMUNICATIONS PROGRAMS

Health communications efforts are a major part of the overall program of health education. It is through effective communication that educators spark interest in their program, convince the target community of the advantages of positive health behaviors, and provide the intellectual foundation for permanent changes. Research suggests that individuals are much more likely to maintain a behavior change when they are aware of the rationale behind it. Effective health communication is an essential part of providing the target community with the skills to maintain positive health changes.

The health communication process has six distinct stages:

- Planning and selecting a strategy: entails analysis of the health issue and the target population; health educators will develop a list of objectives
- Selecting appropriate materials: message format and venue selection
- Developing and pretesting materials: sample of target population is exposed to program; feedback leads to adjustments
- Implementation: program is evaluated and larger changes are considered
- Assessing effectiveness: decision as to whether the goals set in stage 1 are being approached or met
- Feedback to improve program: all pertinent information is reviewed with an eye towards possible changes

COMMUNICATING AND ADVOCATING IN A RANGE OF DIFFERENT SETTINGS

Health educators, in order to be effective, will have to tailor their message for a number of different settings. For example, when making a presentation in a school a health educator will have to take

85

into account the probable indifference of the students; such a presentation will need to be engaging in order to capture the students' interest. When working in a business, on the other hand, a health educator will need to show clients how changes in health behavior will affect them personally. When working in a health care facility, a health educator will have to make sure that his or her message is consistent with the advice of doctors and nurses.

DEVELOPING MATERIAL FOR AN AUDIENCE WITH A LOW READING LEVEL

At all times, a health educator needs to make sure that the information disseminated is simple enough to be understood by the target population. Also, as much as possible the health educators should strive to make written materials interesting and engaging. One way to accomplish these goals is to use everyday vocabulary and call attention to the most important ideas. The basic intent of the text should be summarized at the beginning and end. In some cases, it may be effective to organize the essential points in a bullet format.

SCENARIO ONE

You are a health educator working with a personal care home. You have come across an article which you think might be useful to the residents, but the SMOG test indicates that the article has a ninth-grade readability level.

Explain how you would make the information more accessible to the residents.

The health education information distributed to the general public should be at a fifth or sixth grade reading level. So, if you are given an article which you believe is too sophisticated for your audience, you will need to take steps to simplify it. One way you can do this is by going through and eliminating technical jargon. If the sentences in the article are overly complex, you might simplify them by breaking them up into shorter, smaller sentences. Finally, you might include some accompanying graphics or illustrations that help emphasize the major points of the article.

ASSESSING APPROPRIATE LANGUAGE

Unless the language in health education literature is comprehensible to the target audience, the message will be ineffective. As a general rule, literature to be disseminated to the general public should be composed at a fifth or sixth grade reading level. There should not be any technical jargon, and sentences should be short and direct. Whenever possible, health educators can include graphics and illustrations that support the main points of the text. When there is doubt concerning the acceptability of health literature, there are a number of indices for reading level: Fry Readability scale, SMOG, Fog-Gunning index, and Flesch-Kinkaid, to name a few.

CULTURALLY SENSITIVE COMMUNICATION TECHNIQUES

At all times, a health educator must remain sensitive to the varying cultures and ethnic backgrounds represented in the target community. A health education program cannot contain any elements that prioritize one culture over another, and instructional methods must avoid distinctions based on culture. That being said, it is important to realize that individuals will confront health issues in different ways depending on their cultural background. If you are aware of this and are familiar with cultural characteristics, you can use this to your advantage to create presentations that are engaging and relevant.

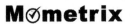

COMMUNICATING HEALTH INFORMATION TO DIFFERENT LEVELS OF SOCIETY

Health educators will have to learn to communicate on the following levels: individual, community, social network, and society. At the individual level, the educator will need to cultivate empathy and respect for the autonomy of each person. At the community level, the educator will need to figure out how best to reach the target audience and design the most useful program of services. When working with social networks, a health educator will be focusing on improving the way in which health-related information is circulated throughout the group. When dealing with health issues as they affect an entire society, a health educator will need to consider how changes in policy and attitude can result in widespread improvements.

ALCOHOL EDUCATION PROGRAMS AIMED AT HIGH SCHOOL SENIORS

There are three professional organizations that you might contact if you are interested in obtaining information about the effectiveness of alcohol education programs for high school seniors:

- American School Health Association (ASHA): Focuses on health education in grades K through 12, particularly the connection between health education and overall academic success
- Society of State Directors of Health, Physical Education, and Recreation (SSDHPER): Composed of state department of education employees; intends to nurture connections between professionals
- Directors of Health Promotion and Education (DHPE): Composed of directors of state-level health programs; aims to help working professionals exchange ideas

PILOT TESTING AND FEEDBACK

Pilot testing typically utilizes the following methods: focus groups, interviews, questionnaires, and readability tests. Pilot testing requires the inclusion of people who possess similar traits/characteristics of the target population. Such people include gatekeepers, opinion leaders, and community influences. CDCynergy has the following steps for pilot testing: test creative concepts with intended audiences to see if ideas resonate, pretest specific messages with intended audiences to ensure that they hear what you want them to, pretest products/materials with intended audiences to ensure they elicit intended response and desired actions, choose pretest settings, and pretest product distribution plans.

INFORMATION AND TECHNOLOGY SKILLS

Information technology is increasingly present in health education, and professionals need to develop some basic skills in this area. For one thing, the use of PowerPoint presentations is ubiquitous in health education, so an aspiring professional had better become fluent in this program. Those professionals who want to make and maintain a decent website will need to learn the basic elements of web design and would do well to learn the techniques for creating and uploading audio and video presentations. Finally, email is the communication method of choice for most professionals these days, so all health educators will need to be conversant with the various email programs and their uses.

MASS MEDIA

Health educators can use the mass media (television, radio, newspapers, magazines, and billboards) to draw attention to a health issue and advocate changes in policy. Of course, success in this endeavor requires a bit of skill. For the most part, mass media advocacy is most effective when it is simple and to the point. Television commercials are not a good venue for highly detailed accounts of health issues. Similarly, drivers can only read so much information off a billboard at one time, so health educators need to be able to condense their message into a few essential words. As much as

87

possible, health educators should strive to make mass media communications lively and engaging, to better draw the interest of a passive public.

The mass media can be an effective venue for health advocacy in some cases. Mass media communications are only effective when they are simplistic, so they should only be used in cases when the health message can be condensed into a few words. Mass media communications are also better at inspiring short term rather than long-term change. For instance, organizing a quick boycott of some unhealthy product would be much easier using mass communication. Mass media communications reach individuals of all intellectual and social levels, so they need to be capable of being understood by as many people as possible.

DECIDING AGAINST USING THE MASS MEDIA

Health educators will probably elect not to use mass media communications to advocate complex changes in health-related behavior or policy. It is simply not effective to expound at length on a health subject in a newspaper advertisement or billboard. When using mass media communications, you need to assume that your audience will only be paying glancing attention. For this reason, you need your message to be succinct and entertaining. Mass media communications are also a bad choice when the health information only applies to a small segment of the population. In this case, it would be more effective to use a communication approach tailored for that specific community.

PLANNING A NEWS CONFERENCE TO INTRODUCE A NEW SCHOOL LUNCH PROGRAM

As a health educator getting ready to introduce a new school lunch program, you might want to send out a news release to generate publicity. This should be done before the school lunch program is introduced. You might also want to invite local journalists to attend the opening day for the new lunch program. Make sure that journalists know when to come and where to go to get good footage for their broadcasts or information for their articles. Many health educators put together information packets and fact sheets for journalists, highlighting the most important points of the new program.

PUBLIC SERVICE ANNOUNCEMENTS

One of the traditional venues through which a health educator can make his or her message known is the public service announcement (PSA). Public service announcements are usually between 15 and 30 seconds long, and therefore need to be direct and succinct. There's not enough time to go into great detail when delivering a public service announcement. Public service announcements are especially useful in delivering one or two pieces of information to a broad audience. They are most effective when they engage the audience and deliver their message with a memorable slogan.

Public Service Announcements must have three common characteristics if they are to be effective. To begin with, a public service announcement must streamline its message. PSAs that speak too broadly will not make any impact; in order to make a strong pitch within the 15 or 30 seconds allotted, the announcement needs to focus on one central issue. It is the job of the health educator to decide which is to be the central issue of the PSA. The second characteristic of an effective PSA is careful production. The images on the screen should support and reinforce the sounds that are coming through the speakers. Finally, an effective PSA will target a very specific contingent. If the audience you are trying to reach is not immediately aware that the PSA concerns them (and them specifically), the message probably will not be received.

TELEVISION

Television is the venue for health communications that will reach the most people. However, television advertisements and public service announcements have obvious time and space constraints, and so are not good at delivering a long and detailed message. Instead, they are appropriate for short, succinct messages that can be whittled down to 1 or 2 main ideas. One disadvantage of using television to disseminate a message is that airtime can be very expensive, especially during peak viewing times. An alternative to paying for airtime is to get booked as a guest on a television talkshow; this is a great way to disseminate a more nuanced message.

RADIO

There are a number of ways that radio can be used to disseminate health information. In the past, health educators have used public service announcements and advertisements to advance their message. Also, health educators have appeared on radio talk shows to promote their agendas. Radio stations often have detailed information about their listening audience, so health educators can be sure to tailor their message appropriately. Unfortunately, radio advertisements and PSAs do not offer enough space to provide a detailed explanation of the health issue.

NEWSPAPERS

Health educators often communicate their message through the newspaper. This can be done in a number of ways. Perhaps the most direct way to spread the word in a newspaper is by writing a letter to the editor. A bit more authority can be achieved by composing an editorial for the paper, although this must be done at the request of the editor. Another way to get newspaper coverage is to hold a press conference and invite newspaper reporters. Print media is perhaps losing some of its popularity, but it is still the best way to distribute detailed information to a large audience.

INTERNET

Health educators are increasingly looking to the Internet as a venue for distributing information. Most health organizations have their own websites, and many individual educators develop blogs or websites that focus on their pet health issues. Health educators can also contribute to chat rooms and newsgroups that focus on health-related issues. The beauty of the Internet is that space is unlimited, so you can go into as much detail as you like. Also, purchasing space on the web is extremely inexpensive. On the other hand, much of the information on the web is unreliable, so you will need to be sure to establish your credentials to your target audience.

NEWS RELEASE

Occasionally, a health educator will need to compose a news release to generate publicity for a special event or incipient health program. A standard news release leads with the most important information and is written in a succinct, terse style. It is important that the news release contains all of the important information, including who is involved in the event, the nature of the event, where will the event be held, and when. A news release should also contain contact information for the organization putting on the event or offering the program. Although news releases are typically written in a dry style, they should include some facts that will generate public interest and encourage the attention of the news media.

It is typical to include the most important information at the beginning of a news release so that the individual at the news organization who reads the release will immediately understand its importance. You do not want to rely on a journalist to read the entire document before deciding whether to publicize your event or program. Also, it is common for media outlets to edit news releases before broadcasting them; you can assist the editing process by including the most vital information at the beginning of the release. In general, you do not want a news release to exceed two or three paragraphs.

ORGANIZATIONAL/COMMUNITY CHANNELS

One common way to disseminate health information in a large group is through organizational or community channels. This might mean holding a town hall meeting, organizing a local conference, or sponsoring a charity event in the neighborhood. Health organizations that make themselves an active contributor to the community are more likely to attract interest from the citizens. This is especially true when the health organization receives the endorsement of respected community leaders. There is a bit of cost associated with using organizational and community channels for communication, but these channels tend to reach a large number of people in a meaningful way.

INTERPERSONAL CHANNELS

One of the best venues for health communication is through interpersonal channels. Studies suggest that individuals are much more receptive to information received through direct, one-on-one communication. This can be in a counseling or consulting setting, or during a conversation on a health hotline. One of the advantages of interpersonal communication is that it gives the client a chance to ask whatever questions are relevant to his or her own situation. On the other hand, one-on-one communication is not a very efficient way to disseminate health information.

When communicating through interpersonal channels, you may want to have brochures or pamphlets for the client to take home and review. It may also be helpful to have some basic guides and graphical depictions to assist your explanation of any complex subjects. When you are conducting a town hall meeting or community conference, you will definitely want to have some graphs and charts, or possibly a PowerPoint presentation, to back up what you are saying. Obviously, when spreading your message through the mass media you will need to have composed a video or audio message for broadcast.

SOCIAL MARKETING AND MARKETING STRATEGIES

Health educators can vastly improve the quality of their health communications programs by incorporating the insights of social marketing. Social marketing is the use of commercial marketing techniques to promote behavior that will improve society. In health education, there is a constant effort to "sell" the benefits of positive health behavior to the members of the target community. Social marketing can be used to introduce a population to a health issue, to increase awareness of health services, or to reinforce positive health behaviors.

8 PS OF THE EXPANDED MARKETING MIX

Marketing strategists often refer to the four Ps of the discipline: product, promotion, place, and price. The branch of marketing known as social marketing, however, requires consideration of four more Ps: publics, partnership, policy advocacy, and purse strings. By "publics," we mean the target audience of the social marketing campaign. An effective campaign will have a well-defined audience and a smart strategy for reaching it. By "partnership," we mean collaborators; an effective social marketing campaign will require participation from respected members of the community. "Policy advocacy" is the effort to promote changes in legislation and organizational policy that will lead to better health behaviors. Finally, by "purse strings" we mean the financial resources that will be required to support the marketing campaign.

Health educators often use the strategies of commercial marketing to communicate important health information to the marketing process. The marketing process has six distinct stages:

- Market analysis: Inventory of data and required resources
- Planning: Establishment of budget, program structure, goals, promotional plan, and schedules
- Developing and testing materials: Program is tested on sample group
- Implementation: Program is applied in its entirety
- Assessing effectiveness: Processes are evaluated according to established indicators
- Feedback for refinement: adjustments made as necessary

In the second stage of the marketing process, health educators will be focused on planning an effective communications program. During this period, they will pay special attention to the so-called "4 Ps" of basic product marketing: product, promotion, place, and price. It is essential to have a well-defined product that is in keeping with the overall goals of the education program. It is also important that the site where this product will be distributed is known and is acceptable. The price of the program must be reasonable given the revenue that can be expected. Finally, the method of promoting the program must be ideal for reaching the target population.

EFFECTIVE EDUCATIONAL MEDIA

There are a number of different types of media that can be effective in disseminating a health-related message. It will be left to the educator to decide which format is most appropriate. For some audiences, as for instance schoolchildren, a video or slide presentation may be the most effective form of communication. For a more sophisticated audience, on the other hand, a detailed piece of health literature might be more appropriate. When dealing with an audience that is not naturally predisposed to take an interest in health matters, the mode of presentation needs to make clear the direct relevance of the health issue in the lives of the audience.

ELECTRONIC COMMUNICATION

Health educators are increasingly turning to electronic media to communicate with the public. One of the great advantages of the Internet for promoting health issues is that subjects can be treated with a great degree of detail, and conversations between educators and constituents are possible. For this reason, many health educators frequently visit health-related websites and chat rooms, where they advocate changes in health policy and try to promote awareness. Also, it is ever easier to include audio and video presentations as part of a website. Really, the only disadvantage of communicating through the electronic media is that Internet access is not ubiquitous in impoverished communities.

ORAL COMMUNICATION

When delivering a speech, a health educator must take care to deliver his or her message clearly and completely. The audience for a speech may not be familiar with the subject, and so the health educator may need to go into some detail to provide background information. Whenever possible, a health educator should include visual representations and graphs to support what he or she is saying. If the speech is being given to a small group, the educator may want to stop occasionally and ask if there are any questions. Oral presentations are not a good venue for complicated, technical explanations; this kind of information is more effectively offered in a written communication.

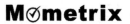

DEVELOPING WRITTEN AND PRINT MATERIALS

Probably the most common method of communication in health education is print media. It is relatively inexpensive to produce and distribute a newsletter or brochure. One common strategy for distribution used by many health organizations is to place the promotional literature in a place where it is likely to be seen by the target population. For instance, it might be a good idea to place brochures on the dangers of smoking on top of a cigarette vending machine. Literature concerning proper nutrition for pregnant mothers could be placed in the waiting room of a gynecologist or obstetrician.

HEALTH COMMUNICATION PROCESS MODEL

The Health Communication Process Model has been developed to streamline the process of distributing health information in a community. It is a computerized template into which educators can enter specifications to determine the precise menu of services and promotional tools that will be most effective. The Health Communication Process Model encourages educators to test their message on a small component of the target population before distributing it to the population at large. The model also helps the educator to compose a rigorous budget outlining the benefits and costs of a given communication program.

BECOMING PROFICIENT IN COMMUNICATING HEALTH INFORMATION

Becoming proficient in health communication is an ongoing process for a health educator. The best way to improve your skills as a communicator is to elicit feedback from the audience. Health organizations often convene focus groups to critique their television and radio advertisements, but even individual educators can ask for audience response after making a presentation or leading a conference. Often, you can elicit more honest responses by having audience members fill out anonymous surveys. Be sure to ask the audience not only whether they enjoyed the presentation, but whether they understood it.

EVALUATING POLICY CHANGE DUE TO ADVOCACY EFFORTS

Savvy health educators will establish benchmarks for assessing the influence that advocacy is having on policy decisions. At the beginning of advocacy efforts, the educator should consider what changes will need to occur in order for advocacy to be considered a success. Note that advocacy can still be considered useful even if it does not result in the precise changes advocated; increasing awareness of a health issue is a positive byproduct of advocacy as well. As the educator leads advocacy efforts, he or she should consider the effectiveness of the strategy and should make any necessary adjustments.

ADVOCACY

Health educators, one way or another, are always advocating for health education. Simply developing and implementing a health education program is a form of advocacy. So, in order to make these advocacy efforts as effective as possible, a health educator should take close consideration of the target audience and the means of presentation. As much as possible, the message should be adapted to the audience. Also, health educators should strive to create conditions in the community that make it receptive to health-related information.

Advocacy in health education is any effort to positively alter policies concerning health. Health educators may advocate changes in the policy of a government, business, or another organization. Effective advocacy requires strong knowledge of the topic in question and a good understanding of how to increase the knowledge of the decision-makers. Legislators and policymakers are typically very busy people, so health educators need to be able to condense their message and deliver it

92

effectively. Health educators need to be able to demonstrate how adjusting a health-related policy will actually be in a policymaker's own interests.

Advocacy is the pursuit of influencing outcomes, including public policy and resource allocation decisions within political, economic, and social systems and institutions that directly affect people's lives. Health information needs are based upon acknowledging the factors that influence and pertain to health status such as medical care, public health, social behavior, and the environment. Issues that may influence health and health education need to be identified, and there are multiple possible sources of advocacy for such issues. Some sources of advocacy include peer-reviewed journals, federal websites, Health Education Associations, and national non-governmental organizations.

Effective advocacy can be accomplished even by individuals. The best way for an individual to advocate is to become informed on a health issue and then write letters to his or her government representatives. Individuals can also help promote positive changes in health behavior by setting a good example, educating their peers on health topics, and participating in promotional events. Individuals can also advocate positive changes in health policy by writing editorials and letters to the editor of a newspaper or magazine.

It is important to engage stakeholders in advocacy by developing a careful advocacy plan. The advocacy plan should include the following: goals, organizational considerations, constituents, allies, opponents, targets, and tactics. It is essential to remember advocacy initiatives when engaging stakeholders. Advocacy initiatives are designed to influence policy and law, often include activities such as education, lobbying, and mobilization. Stakeholders should be involved in leading advocacy initiatives by understanding the priority of the key issues in public health and education, helping to identify useful social networks, fundraising, and participation in strategic planning.

When developing an advocacy plan, it is important to comply with current local, state, and federal policies and procedures. The following are forces that impact health-related policies: the United States Congress, the Federal Health Agencies, states, health care providers, businesses, and local communities. Prior to focusing upon legislative advocacy, it is essential to consider the following factors in the development of health policy development: needs assessment of the community, scientific analysis of the results, the impact of any current programs, and the availability of resources that will be used to support and maintain the policy.

The two most important factors that make advocacy effective are knowledge and planning. In order to be an effective advocate, a health educator has to fully understand the problem as well as its potential solutions. The health educator also has to understand how best to present this information to those individuals or organizations that can make positive changes. Health educators also have to be good at planning in order to be effective advocates. This involves laying out an organized plan for lobbying lawmakers and policymakers, and then marshaling appropriate resources until the proposed changes have been made.

There are many advocacy strategies, such as voting behavior, electioneering, direct lobbying, grassroots lobbying, Internet use to obtain health information, and media advocacy. Media advocacy is a strong tool for the certified health education specialist to use when developing an advocacy plan. The following questions should be addressed when using media advocacy in the development of an advocacy plan: What is the problem? What is the solution? Who will support the solution? What needs to be said and how to gain attention? It is also vital to remember that national health policies will help prioritize advocacy.

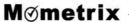

GETTING CITIZENS INVOLVED IN THE HEALTH-DECISION-MAKING PROCESS

There are four basic ways that a health educator can involve citizens in the process of making health decisions:

- Make sure the health program affects all members of the community: Citizens will not be likely to get involved unless they see themselves as stakeholders
- Ask for feedback: Most people will be flattered if you ask them for advice and comments on a new program
- Establish a clear system for getting involved: Too many programs are underpatronized simply because they fail to lay out the specific steps for participation
- Emphasize the role of community involvement: Program plans should include attention to the importance of community involvement

HEALTH POLICY

Health policy originates in a number of different places. The health policies administered by the federal government are the results of legislation passed by the members of Congress and authorized by the President. Some health policies will be terminated or modified based on the decisions of the judicial system. In a business, health policies are developed by the management in accordance with all pertinent legislation. In a community, however, health policy may be a much more free-form topic. Health educators can practice advocacy to improve health policy in all of these venues.

POLICY ANALYSIS

It is important for the certified health education specialist to proactively analyze and assemble data in order to ensure evidence is ready when a policy window/opportunity opens. The data should demonstrate the following when used in policy analysis: burden on the health of the public, priority over other issues, pertinence at the local level, interventional benefits, personalization of the issue by using vignettes/stories about how lives are impacted, and the estimated interventional costs. Policy analysis and research findings should be utilized for information in health policy debates and to provide information for policy makers.

EVIDENCE-BASED RESEARCH AND DECISION-MAKING

Evidence-based research is a type of research in which the researcher is aware of certain evidence before exploring the subject. In short, the researcher does not enter the project unbiased; he or she is aware of a theory derived from the evidence and uses research to test its validity. One of the reasons to utilize evidence-based research to develop policies to promote health is that such usage ensures that the researcher has been working with established studies and prior research. Using established theories is also cost-effective since it obviates the necessity of starting from scratch.

When policymakers refer to evidence-based decision-making, they mean that choices are not made until a careful, objective scrutiny of hard data has been performed. Policymakers who practice evidence-based decision-making will need to see hard evidence before they are willing to come to any conclusions. As a health educator, you will need to be skilled at assembling inventories of hard data to support your program or policy. For example, if you are advocating the elimination of smoking in restaurants, you had better provide data suggesting the health risks of second-hand smoke. It is not enough to merely state that tobacco smoke is unpleasant and sticks to the clothing.

STATE-OF-THE-ART HEALTH EDUCATION PRACTICE

State-of-the-art health education practice involves multiple elements, such as the focus on definitive health goals and the concomitant outcomes in behavior. Another aspect is that the health education

94

is research-based and theory-driven. Health education practice addresses individual values and group norms that support health-enhancing behaviors. Another important aspect of health education is the focus on increasing personal perception of risk and harmfulness of engaging in specific health risk behaviors and reinforcing protective factors. A vital element in health education is to focus on social pressures and peer influences. Another focus is on that of building individual competence.

INFLUENCING DECISION MAKERS

Health educators will need to rely on a varied repertoire of techniques for influencing policy decision-makers. The most important thing is to know the mind of the decision-maker in question. If you can understand the interests and values of the individual you are trying to influence, you will most likely understand how best to appeal to this person. For instance, some decision-makers will be disciples of hard data; they will not respond to any arguments that are not supported by clear statistical proof. Other individuals will be more susceptible to emotional appeals and anecdotal evidence. Still others can only be moved to change when they are shown how it is in their self-interest.

POLICY ADVOCACY

Policy advocacy is the effort of individuals and organizations to persuade the government to improve its health policies. Policy advocacy can be performed by individuals, organizations, or coalitions. Some of the common techniques of policy advocacy are petitions, letter-writing campaigns, and public service announcements. In some cases, and especially before an election, policy advocates will circulate information among voters.

Advocacy on health issues is not limited to lobbyists and bureaucrats; indeed, every health educator should do as much as possible to improve public awareness and legislative policy related to health issues. One easy way to advocate changes in health policy is to write or call a government official or policymaker. Another is to disseminate health information to influential individuals. Health educators can also write editorials and letters to the editor. In order to be an effective advocate on health issues, it is important to keep abreast of all relevant research.

MEDIA ADVOCACY

Media advocacy is the effort to use media exposure to generate support for a change in health policy. Health educators often write editorials or letters to the editor of a newspaper or magazine in an effort to win recognition for a particular cause. Organizations may hold press conferences or produce public service announcements as a way of promoting changes in health policy. Media advocacy is more appropriate for simple messages that can be described in a short format. Also, media advocacy efforts need to be composed at a level that can be understood by non-experts.

LEGISLATIVE ADVOCACY

Legislative advocacy is simply the branch of health advocacy wherein educators work with lawmakers to make positive changes in government health policy. Legislative advocacy can be practiced as an individual by contacting state and federal representatives. Most health organizations, however, employ special lobbyists to promote their interests in Washington. One of the goals of these organizations is to provide politicians with the facts to make informed decisions. One example of legislative advocacy might be telling politicians about the dangers of a certain kind of insulation, in the hopes that they will ban this product from being sold.

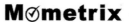

RESPONSIBILITY TO PROMOTE THE HEALTH EDUCATION PROFESSION

A certified health education specialist has a responsibility to promote the health education profession and to communicate the role of the profession in implementing, evaluating, translating, and disseminating effective health education and promotion practices. The seven areas of responsibility are as follows: assess needs, assets, and capacity for health education; plan health education; implement health education; conduct evaluation and research related to health education; administer and manage health education; serve as a health education resource person; and communicate and advocate for health and health education.

PRIMARY FUNCTION OF A HEALTH EDUCATOR

Health educators are charged with informing the public about how to lead a healthier life. In order to do this, a health educator will plan and implement programs targeted with encouraging specific behavioral changes. At different times, a health educator will have to use a number of different pedagogical methods. In order to be successful, a health educator will have to encourage the target population to agree with the premises of the program. A health educator will also have to be able to marshal the necessary resources to accomplish the program goals. He or she will have to plan program activities and put them into action. Perhaps most importantly, a health educator will have to establish a system for monitoring the progress of the program.

BRIEF DESCRIPTION OF PROFESSIONAL ASSOCIATIONS FOR HEALTH EDUCATORS

- DHPE: Directors of Health Promotion and Education; group of departmental directors that seeks to increase advocacy, training, and resource accumulation for health projects
- SOPHE: Society for Public Health Education; focuses on public health advocacy and professional development
- SSDHER: Society of State Directors of Health, Physical Education, and Recreation; state officials responsible for monitoring health and physical education programs in public schools
- CNHEO: Coalition of National Health Education Organizations; fosters connections between nine public health professional organizations
- AAHE: American Association for Health Education; affiliated with the American Alliance for Health, Physical Education, Recreation, and Dance; aims to assist health educators' efforts to promote wellness in all difference environments
- ACHA: American College Health Association; a group of academic professionals devoted to the promotion of wellness
- APHA: American Public Health Association; group of researchers and health professionals devoted to preventing disease
- ASHA: American School Health Association; education professionals who seek to promote health education in the K-12 setting
- Eta Sigma Gamma: the national health education honorary that seeks to promote high professional standards among health educators

DHPE (ASTDHPPHE)

The DHPE (or ASTDHPPHE, standing for Association of State and Territorial Directors of Health Promotion and Public Health Education) is composed of directors of health education and health promotion departments in the United States. This organization exists primarily as a venue for communications between directors of various health programs. The organization believes that the profession is strengthened when directors can share their experience. Specifically, the DHPE focuses on training, fundraising, and policy efforts. It also publishes a journal called *The Voice*.

SOPHE (Society for Public Health Education)

The SOPHE (Society for Public Health Education) is composed of health education professionals and health education students. It was originally formed in 1950. SOPHE focuses on advocacy on public health issues and professional development. One of the ways that SOPHE promotes professional development is by sponsoring continuing education programs for health professionals. SOPHE publishes the journals *Health Education and Behavior* and *Health Promotion Practice* and the newsletter *News and Views*.

SSDHPER (Society of State Directors of Health, Physical Education, and Recreation)

The SSDHPER (Society of State Directors of Health, Physical Education, and Recreation) is composed of the individuals who direct health and physical education programs for state departments of education. The organization exists to connect professionals and advocate positive changes in state and national policy. It is very common for the SSDHPER to partner with the DHPE to achieve a common goal. The organization also promotes professional development by offering training and workshops for students. The SSDHER publishes a newsletter called *The Society Page*.

CNHEO (Coalition of National Health Education Organizations)

The CNHEO (Coalition of National Health Education Organizations) is composed of the members of nine other health professional organizations, including the American Association for Health Education, the American School Health Association, and the Society for Public Health Education. This coalition aims to use its combined strength to make positive changes in health education policy. The delegates of the coalition give advice to the member organizations and advocate policy changes in Washington.

AAHE (American Association for Health Education)

The AAHE (American Association for Health Education) is a subsidiary of the American Alliance for Health, Physical Education, Recreation, and Dance. This organization aims to assist educators specializing in physical education, leisure, fitness, dance, health promotion, and education. The organization employs a number of lobbyists in Washington, who work to influence policy in favor of educators. In particular, the AAHE works to establish systematic health programs in schools, colleges, businesses, and other organizations. The organization also publishes the *Journal of Health Education* and the newsletter *HExtra*.

ACHA (American College Health Association

The ACHA (American College Health Association) consists of university-level educators in health and fitness. These individuals may be professors, doctors, nurses, and students. The purpose of this organization is to promote awareness and positive health behaviors on campus. The ACHA publishes the Journal of American College Health. At present, it is affiliated with approximately 1000 institutions and has 2500 individual members.

APHA (American Public Health Association)

The APHA (American Public Health Association) is the longest-running public health organization in the United States; it has been around since the 19th century. It consists of a coalition of researchers and other public-health professionals; the purpose of the organization is to prevent disease through advocacy (by its Public Health Education and Promotion Section) and education (by its School Health Education and Services Section). The APHA also publishes the *American Journal of Public Health* and a newsletter called *The Nation's Health*.

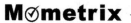

ASHA (AMERICAN SCHOOL HEALTH ASSOCIATION)

The ASHA (American School Health Association, formerly known as the American Association of School Physicians) is composed of health professionals with an interest in K-12 health education. The organization declares that its mission is to promote and support school health programs by providing financial assistance and other resources. The organization also supports health teacher training. The ASHA publishes the *Journal of School Health* and the newsletter *Pulse*.

ETA SIGMA GAMMA

Eta Sigma Gamma is the national education honorary, meaning that it bestows numerous awards for individuals who raise the profile of the health education profession. The organization was originally developed to promote professional development and raise standards among health professionals. It has its headquarters at Ball State University in Muncie, Indiana. Eta Sigma Gamma publishes two journals, the *Health Educator* and *The Health Education Monograph Series*, and a newsletter, *Vision*.

AAHB (AMERICAN ACADEMY OF HEALTH BEHAVIOR)

The AAHB (American Academy of Health Behavior) is composed of health behavior scholars. Its intent is to strengthen the research foundation of the health education profession and encourage the application of research to professional practice. It also seeks to publicize what it considers to be important research findings. One of its other purposes is to facilitate communication between research scholars in various fields. The AAHB publishes the *American Journal of Health Behavior*.

PROFESSIONAL PREPARATION

The goals of the health educator and professional preparation are as follows: recruit and train grassroots educators, strengthen mentoring of young professionals, identify strategies to draw students to the profession, standardize accreditation of programs, provide certification and increase the number of Certified Health Education Specialists, provide in-service training/continuing education for health education professionals on emerging technology, establish mentoring programs, reinforce pride and commitment in professional preparation and encourage active involvement in professional associations, adapt curricula according to the evolution of the field and the world, standardize the practice of the profession, and educate about technology.

PROFESSIONAL GROWTH

There are a number of certification and licensing programs that indicate professional progress on the part of a health educator. Many health educators will be required to become Certified Health Education Specialists. Those who do will have to complete 75 continuing education contact hours in order to maintain this certification. To maintain certification, a Certified Health Education Specialist will need to stay abreast of professional literature, attend conferences, and publish journal articles. Some health educators will obtain master's degrees in their area of specialization.

Every health educator should develop a personal plan for professional growth, as a means of keeping themselves on track. Professional growth should include program-centered goals as well as individual goals. For instance, a health educator should try to accumulate as many distinct skills as possible and should take definite steps to improve his or her performance in developing, implementing, and communicating in health programs. If the health educator is focused on a particular area of practice, as for instance in businesses or schools, he or she may have specific professional goals related to this setting.

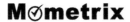

CREDENTIALING AND QUALITY ASSURANCE

The role of credentialing serves an integral purpose in assuring the integrity and the quality assurance of the health education profession. The goals of quality assurance and credentialing are to standardize professional practice, require credentialing nationally to practice, and have it specified in job descriptions (Certified Health Education Specialist preferred) under "required knowledge, abilities, and skills." Other goals are to include health education competencies in standardized assessments in recruitment and retention, and in requirements and guidelines for jobs; develop and model standards for health education programs; publicize the code of ethics; and participate in review boards.

HISTORY OF THE HEALTH EDUCATION PROFESSION

One of the most significant aspects in the history of the health education profession was the accreditation of schools and programs that offered degrees with a concentration in health education and the establishment of a credentialing system for health educators. Other key aspects in the history of the health education profession include health education standards for school programs and students, and the development of common definitions for important concepts in health education. In 1995, the National Commission for Health Education Credentialing, Inc., and the Coalition of National Health Education Organizations, USA, had a forum to work on the future of health education.

The 1995 forum that was convened in Atlanta, Georgia, served to focus on the future of the health education profession. One of the goals of the forum was to define and to achieve goals and objectives intended to advance the profession of health education and to speak with a common voice on issues affecting the profession. One of the outcomes of the 1995 forum led to six focal areas to serve as guides to advance health education. The six areas are professional preparation, quality assurance, research, advocacy, promoting the profession, and dynamic/contemporary practice.

Practice Test

1. Which of the following is a secondary intervention aimed at preventing communicable disease in a priority population?

    a. Chlorination of the water supply
    b. Quarantining children infected with measles
    c. Immunization program
    d. Post-meningitis rehabilitation program

2. A staff member in a health education program to increase HIV/AIDS testing and safe sex practices among gay males in an inner city posted personal information about one client (although not the person's name) on a social media site. This is a violation of which ethical principle?

    a. Confidentiality
    b. Privacy
    c. Nonmaleficence
    d. Justice

3. If the health education specialist is planning a class exercise in which the class members will need to work in small groups, what is most likely to be the best room seating arrangement?

    a. Circle
    b. Half-circle
    c. Cluster
    d. U-seating

4. If the health education specialist is engaged in a campaign to encourage employees at a large company to have flu shots as one method to decrease seasonal absenteeism, the best strategy for gaining attention about the issue is probably

    a. emails.
    b. newsletters.
    c. posters.
    d. paycheck stuffers.

5. If the health education specialist wants visual data to show health care trends regarding healthcare quality and disparities in order to justify a program, the best source is probably

    a. CDC.
    b. AHRQ.
    c. PubMed/MEDLINE.
    d. the Cochrane Library.

6. When the health education specialist explains why technology resources benefit the priority population, the health education specialist is applying the ethical principle of

    a. justice.
    b. veracity.
    c. beneficence.
    d. nonmaleficence

7. The health education specialist is implementing a diabetic clinic as part of a health education program to decrease rates of diabetes and diabetic complications among a priority population comprised primarily of undocumented Mexican immigrants with no insurance; however, only a few people have used the clinic because of fears about deportation. What is most likely to be the best marketing plan?

  a. Targeted mailing in Spanish to members of the priority population
  b. Gaining support of key informants in the community
  c. Ads in local Spanish language newspapers
  d. Billboards marketing the program in the community

8. In order to assess progress in achieving objectives, the health education specialist must first determine

  a. indicators.
  b. methods.
  c. responsibility.
  d. costs.

9. Utilizing the social analysis network tool PARTNER (Program to Analyze, Record, and Track Networks to Enhance Relationship) to monitor a partnership allows the health education specialist to (1) create visuals showing connections, (2) assess network scores, and (3) assess

  a. timeline.
  b. gaps in processes.
  c. outcomes measures.
  d. financial reports.

10. If the health education specialist working for a nonprofit healthcare organization needs to present the results of data collection to the board of directors of the organization, what is the best way to present the data?

  a. Charts and raw data
  b. Summarize verbally
  c. Charts only
  d. Raw data only

11. When applying Bridge's Transition Model to help people in an organization cope with change in the initial stage when they are uncomfortable and/or resistant to change, the health education specialist should

  a. ignore resistance and appear positive.
  b. support people and provide guidance.
  c. celebrate change, reward people, and commit to change.
  d. listen to people and communicate.

12. If members of a priority population take exercise classes and participate in smoking cessation programs, the need for these services would be classified as

  a. perceived.
  b. expressed.
  c. normative.
  d. actual.

13. The first step in the marketing process to facilitate change is to

    a. analyze the situation.
    b. determine the role of marketing.
    c. select goals and objectives.
    d. Select priority populations.

14. The health education specialist has developed a new protocol and tools for teaching new parents to properly care for infants. Before implementing the program, the health education specialist should

    a. survey staff.
    b. determine problems.
    c. carry out pilot testing.
    d. conduct further research.

15. The health education specialist has received a notice from a community foundation that, because of an increase in funding for another agency and decreased revenue, an anticipated grant cannot be provided to implement the program the health education specialist has developed. The first step in dealing with this barrier to implementation should be to

    a. delay implementation of the program.
    b. search for alternative funding sources.
    c. appeal to the community foundation to reconsider.
    d. modify the program to decrease costs.

16. When utilizing data mining as part of data collection, data mining is used primarily for

    a. descriptive analysis.
    b. prescriptive analysis.
    c. inferential analysis.
    d. predictive analysis.

17. When using the Ecological Systems Model to assess the capacity of stakeholders to meet program goals, the health education specialist should recognize that

    a. multiple factors affect behavior.
    b. influences on behavior act independently on the individual.
    c. usually one primary factor affects behavior.
    d. behavior is unrelated to physical and sociocultural surroundings.

18. The health education specialist is advocating for a free clinic to serve the homeless population as well as undocumented immigrants. All of the following are efforts that may engage stakeholders in the advocacy efforts EXCEPT

    a. focus groups to review plans for the clinic.
    b. interview with key informants to discuss plans.
    c. publicly criticizing the community for inaction.
    d. conducting surveys regarding location of the clinic.

19. The health education specialist carries out a community needs assessment as part of a public health program. The needs assessment shows a markedly increased rate of HIV among injection drug users because of increased heroin use and needle sharing. An example of an appropriate outcome based on this assessment is

    a. elimination of new HIV infections in the community.

    b. elimination of injection drug use.

    c. increased punishment for drug dealers.

    d. establishment of a needle exchange program.

20. The health education specialist carries out a community needs assessment as part of a public health program. The needs assessment shows a markedly increased rate of HIV among injection drug users because of increased heroin use and needle sharing. If the health education specialist commits the public health department to work with another community agency to promote the common goal of reducing HIV infections related to injection drug use, what type of intervention the health education specialist is utilizing?

    a. Consultation

    b. Collaboration

    c. Advocacy

    d. Outreach

21. Which of the following is most likely to be the impact of a strictly enforced local ordinance against sleeping on the streets or in the parks overnight in the downtown area in order to remove the homeless?

    a. Increased numbers of shelters

    b. Shift of homeless population to outside the downtown area

    c. Decrease in the homeless population of the area

    d. Increase in crimes against property

22. Which of the following is an example of a voluntary health agency with which the health education specialist may collaborate in carrying out preventive health projects?

    a. Ford Foundation

    b. Shriner's

    c. American Heart Association

    d. The American Academy of Health Behavior

23. When storing and utilizing large amounts of personal data about members of a priority population, what is the primary concern?

    a. Accuracy

    b. Ease of access

    c. Clarity

    d. Security

24. Which step in media literacy is the health education specialist utilizing when using media devices to convene a priority population?

    a. Reaction

    b. Awareness

    c. Reflection

    d. Analysis

25. When considering the best method of surveying a population for a needs assessment, what is the first thing to consider?

    a. Resources needed for assessment
    b. Timeframe required for assessment
    c. Characteristics of the target population
    d. Ease of administration of assessment

26. The health education specialist plans to conduct community forums and to interview key informants regarding needs of a priority population for health-related information. Prior to the forums and interviews, the health education specialist should

    a. draw up a list of suggestions.
    b. review literature and social indicators.
    c. ask for volunteers to disseminate health information.
    d. form focus groups to discuss needs.

27. If a television ad for a health campaign has a large reach but a poor recall, the problem is probably

    a. hour of viewing.
    b. size of audience.
    c. presentation of material.
    d. audience literacy.

28. The health education specialist is concerned about healthcare disparities and wants to participation in advocacy efforts. The health education specialist's advocacy efforts should begin with

    a. local public health department.
    b. personal practice.
    c. state legislature.
    d. federal legislature.

29. The health education specialist has placed information about the need for vaccinations on a kiosk in a local mall. What type of communication channel is the health education specialist utilizing?

    a. Community
    b. Interpersonal
    c. Mass media
    d. Organizational

30. When prioritizing community needs for preventive efforts, the three primary considerations are (1) leading causes of death/morbidity, (2) years of potential life lost, and (3)

    a. political support.
    b. population characteristics.
    c. policy.
    d. economic costs.

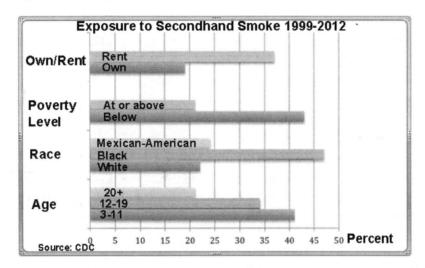

31. Based on the information in the graph above, which two factors are most critical in determining exposure to second-hand smoke?

    a. Poverty level and race
    b. Race and age
    c. Home ownership and age
    d. Poverty level and home ownership

32. When conducting a culture audit of an organization, which finding would be cause for most concern?

    a. Organization employees feel their salaries are too low.
    b. There is some differences of opinion about the vision and mission.
    c. Employees readily identify key decision-makers.
    d. Organization employees are afraid to give their opinions.

33. According to Kotter's 8-Step Change Model, what percentage of key staff should the health education specialist convince that organizational change is warranted?

    a. 25%
    b. 50%
    c. 75%
    d. 100%

34. If a public health organization is utilizing the Six Sigma model for program improvement, the health education specialist should expect much emphasis to be placed on

    a. data collection.
    b. customer satisfaction.
    c. program effectiveness.
    d. cost-effectiveness.

35. The health education specialist is planning to speak to a number of community groups about the importance of HPV vaccinations in an area in which HPV vaccination rates are low because of concerns that the vaccination will encourage promiscuity. Based on these factors, the primary focus of the presentations should probably be on

a. preventing HPV infections.
b. preventing cervical and penile cancer.
c. local sexually-transmitted disease rates.
d. complications of HPV infections.

36. Starting a petition in support of an initiative to increase funding for homeless shelters is an example of what type of advocacy strategy?

a. Electioneering
b. Direct lobbying
c. Grassroots lobbying
d. Media advocacy

37. The health education specialist has developed a Facebook page and Twitter account in order to use social media to reach people in the community. The Facebook page has approximately 3500 followers. How many times per month should the health education specialist plan on updating the Facebook page with new information?

a. More than 60 times
b. 30 to 60 times
c. 10 to 30 times
d. 1 to 5 times

38. A coalition of community agencies has come together to develop a plan to promote a reduction in obesity through healthier lifestyle choices. The next step should be to

a. begin the planning process.
b. establish a timeline.
c. elicit community input regarding the plan.
d. determine the roles of members.

39. When recruiting volunteers to help with implementation of a program, the most important criterion should be

a. skills.
b. motivation.
c. personality.
d. available time.

40. In a needs assessment, *capacity* refers to

a. costs.
b. assets.
c. participants.
d. program reach.

41. An organization's mission statement should include the

    a. identified problems.
    b. organizational structure.
    c. desired outcomes.
    d. organization's purpose.

42. If a community needs assessment is based on results of an Internet survey only, the ethical principle that may be violated is

    a. equity.
    b. veracity.
    c. beneficence.
    d. autonomy.

Questions 43 and 44 pertain to the following graph:

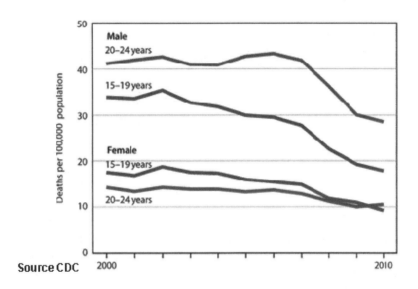

43. According to the graph above, which group showed an increase in motor vehicle-related deaths from 2009 to 2010?

    a. Males 20 to 24 years
    b. Males 15 to 19 years
    c. Females 15 to 19 years
    d. Females 20 to 24 years

44. Based on the information in the graph above, which group would most benefit from a targeted education program regarding motor-vehicle safety?

    a. Males 20 to 24 years
    b. Males 15 to 19 years
    c. Females 15 to 19 years
    d. Females 20 to 24 years

45. The National Task Force on the Preparation and Practice of Health Educators was first established in what year?

    a. 1970
    b. 1978
    c. 1985
    d. 1990

46. If searching for statistics regarding rates of tuberculosis, which of the following is an appropriate source of secondary data?

    a. OSHA
    b. Census Bureau
    c. CDC
    d. CMS

47. If two organizations have agreed to collaborate on an educational program as separate entities with no sharing of financial resources and each organization carrying out different functions, the organizations should likely have a

    a. contract.
    b. memorandum of understanding.
    c. letter of intent.
    d. partnership agreement.

48. If utilizing a logic model to show how a program aligns with the mission and goals of an organization, the health education specialist would typically develop a flowchart with at least three categories: input, output, and

    a. outcomes.
    b. goals.
    c. costs.
    d. gaps.

49. The health education specialist is assessing the potential use of the smart watch, such as the Apple Watch, and software applications to remotely monitor the vital signs and exercise of participants in a health improvement program. The primary concern about using this new technology is likely

    a. ease of use.
    b. cost.
    c. invasion of privacy.
    d. maintenance.

50. If the health education specialist plans to present the rationale for a community program to a coalition of community agencies and organizations that meet monthly, the best method of communication is probably a(n)

    a. written report submitted to the monthly meeting.
    b. telephone call to key members.
    c. oral presentation at the monthly meeting.
    d. email to all members of the coalition.

51. Following a small successful pilot test, the county health department has decided to implement a smoking cessation program throughout the widespread county, including a city with a large diverse population and outlying suburbs, towns, and rural areas. The best method for implementation is probably

    a. phased-in implementation by location.
    b. phased in implementation by population groups.
    c. full implementation.
    d. large-scale pilot test.

52. A health education specialist working for a large business wants to develop a multifaceted fitness program for employees but must secure resources through a request to top management. When preparing the presentation, the health education specialist should focus on

    a. benefits to the business.
    b. benefits to the employees.
    c. resources needed to implement the program.
    d. health education specialist's role.

53. If the health education specialist hires a consultant to install hardware and software as part of program implementation, the health education specialist should prepare a(n)

    a. list of tasks.
    b. memorandum of understanding.
    c. interagency cooperation contract.
    d. statement of work (SOW).

Questions 54 and 55 pertain to the following graph:

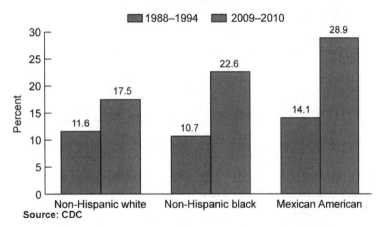

Prevalence of obesity among boys aged 12–19 years, by race and ethnicity: United States, 1988–1994 and 2009–2010

Source: CDC

54. Based on the national statistics in the graph above, which ethnic group of boys 12 to 19 showed the greatest increase in obesity between 1994 and 2009?

    a. Data inconclusive
    b. Non-Hispanic whites
    c. Non-Hispanic blacks
    d. Mexican Americans

55. Considering the information in the graph above, what is the next step to take if developing a program to fight adolescent obesity?

a. Target the group with the greatest increase in obesity.
b. Obtain local statistics about adolescent obesity.
c. Target all adolescent groups, regardless of ethnicity.
d. Survey the community to determine interest in a program.

56. Which of the following is NOT an appropriate question to ask during the first step of a needs assessment?

a. "What is the goal of the needs assessment?"
b. "What resources are needed for the assessment?"
c. "What interventions should be instituted?"
d. "How extensive should the needs assessment be?"

57. When extracting data from a database using Boolean operators, if the health education specialist wants to retrieve documents that contain information about hypertension associated with obesity among adolescent African Americans, the most appropriate search is

a. hypertension and obesity and adolescent and African American.
b. hypertension or obesity and adolescent or African American.
c. hypertension or obesity or adolescent or African American.
d. hypertension or obesity and adolescent and African American not Caucasian.

58. The first issue to consider when determining the validity of data is the

a. exclusion criteria.
b. inclusion criteria.
c. date.
d. source.

59. If the health education specialist conducted a survey to determine how many employees smoke in the workplace but wants more information about smoking behavior, the best method for data collection is probably

a. focus groups.
b. observation.
c. nominal group process.
d. Delphi panel.

60. All of the following are reasons to train personnel who are assisting with data collection EXCEPT

a. to prevent ethics violations.
b. to ensure timely collection.
c. to ensure consistency.
d. to guarantee accurate analysis.

61. The primary problem with using only community forums to gather data about a priority population is that

a. the forum members may not be representative of the population.
b. community forums may be too time-consuming.
c. locating a place to hold community forums is difficult.
d. community forums are expensive to hold.

62. A state with a large undocumented immigrant population has prohibited the use of public funds to provide healthcare for this population. The impact of this legislation is likely

a. decreased population of undocumented immigrants.
b. increased disease and disability.
c. increased crime rates.
d. increased number of free clinics.

63. If the health education specialist is interested in conducting legislative lobbying about a number of health-related issues, the health education specialist should begin by

a. telephoning as many legislators as possible.
b. focusing on one issue.
c. gaining allies.
d. starting on online petition for change.

64. According to the Joint Committee on Standards for Educational Evaluation, the standard that means that information gathered in evaluation must serve the needs of those who will use the information is

a. feasibility.
b. propriety.
c. utility.
d. accuracy.

65. The purpose of using an *outcome chain* is to

a. indicate responsibility for different aspect of assessment.
b. help identify long and short-term outcomes leading to attainment of goals.
c. determine costs of each aspect of assessment.
d. show how activities relate to goal attainment.

66. The local school district has had a high percentage of adolescents diagnosed with sexually transmitted diseases for the past 5 years. The health education specialist is implementing an education program about STDs. The health education specialist has set a goal that within one year there will be no further cases of STDs among adolescents in the school district. What potential problem may arise with this goal?

a. The term *adolescent* is too vague.
b. The goal is unrealistic.
c. The time period is too short.
d. STDs are not clearly defined.

67. The local school district has had a high percentage of adolescents diagnosed with sexually transmitted diseases for the past 5 years. The health education specialist is implementing an education program about STDs. If the health education specialist needs more information about the sexual activity of the adolescents in the school district in order to better plan program strategies, the best method to obtain this information is probably

a. in-class anonymous surveys.
b. mailed anonymous surveys.
c. focus group.
d. student-led discussion groups.

68. The local school district has had a high percentage of adolescents diagnosed with sexually transmitted diseases for the past 5 years. The health education specialist is implementing an education program about STDs. If the health education specialist is planning a delivery method to educate adolescents about the dangers of unprotected sexual activity and different types of sexually transmitted diseases, the best method of delivery is probably a(n)

a. computer video game.
b. computer-assisted instruction module.
c. video presentation.
d. handouts/posters.

69. Which of the following tools is often used to obtain qualitative statistics?

a. State reports
b. Questionnaires
c. Public forums
d. National statistics

70. If using the FOG index to assess readability so that material can be adapted for consumers, what should the health education specialist count first?

a. Number of syllables in a sentence
b. Number of words and sentences in a passage
c. Number of syllables in a passage
d. Number of words with 3 or more syllables

71. The best use of a focus group is to

a. suggest interventions for a population.
b. identify a priority population.
c. carry out a needs assessment.
d. provide a response to proposed interventions.

72. According to *Healthy People 2020*, one aspect of the key area *social and communication context* of social determinants is

a. incarceration/institutionalization.
b. access to health care.
c. crime and violence.
d. quality housing.

73. Which of the following is an example of a societal factor that is considered a root cause of racial and ethnic disparities?

a. Unsafe social environment
b. Health illiteracy
c. Sedentary lifestyle
d. Lack of quality healthcare

74. Which of the following is part of the community level of influence of health behaviors?

a. Knowledge and beliefs
b. Association with family and friends
c. Social networks
d. Rules, regulations, and policies

75. When planning interventions for a priority population in which the eldest male in the family makes the decisions, the health education specialist determines that this method of decision making is counter to American ideals and plans to focus on empowering the women in the population to make independent decisions. This is an example of

    a. cultural blindness.
    b. cultural awareness.
    c. ethnocentrism.
    d. ethnic inequality.

76. When designing interventions for a health promotion, the health education specialist plans a multi-level approach in order to allow any member of the priority population who wants to participate the opportunity to do so. The ethical principle that the health education is applying to this strategy is

    a. beneficence.
    b. veracity.
    c. autonomy.
    d. equity.

77. If using the PRECEDE-PROCEED planning model to guide the delivery of a health promotion plan, which of the following is completed in phase 4, the first phase of the PROCEED portion?

    a. Implementation
    b. Process evaluation
    c. Administrative and policy assessment
    d. Impact evaluation

78. The resources necessary to achieve the objectives of an educational program include those that are human, tangible, and intangible. An example of an intangible resource for an organization is

    a. organization's image.
    b. staff members.
    c. computers.
    d. office space.

79. The time estimates utilized in a Program Evaluation and Review Technique (PERT) chart include all of the following except

    a. optimistic time.
    b. anticipated time.
    c. expected time
    d. pessimistic time.

80. If soliciting feedback about an educational program, the method that will likely provide the best response rate is

    a. emailing surveys to participants at completion of the program.
    b. mailing surveys to participants at completion of the program.
    c. providing printed surveys directly to participants during the program.
    d. asking participants how they feel during the program.

81. The primary purpose of carrying out a feasibility study is to

a. identify factors that may interfere with implementation.
b. assure the program meets the needs of participants.
c. determine cost-effectiveness.
d. identify resources and funding sources.

82. All of the following are sections of Article V, Responsibility in Research and Evaluation, of the Code of Ethics for the Health Education Profession EXCEPT

a. research and Evaluation should do no harm to individuals.
b. participation is voluntary.
c. conflicts of interest are openly shared.
d. education is free from discrimination and harassment.

83. When communicating findings to partners and stakeholders through a written report, in which section should the data analysis plan be described?

a. Introduction
b. Methodology
c. Results
d. Conclusion

84. A health impact assessment (HIA) should generally be carried out

a. before and after development or implementation.
b. after development or implementation.
c. before development or implementation.
d. during development or implementation.

85. If findings of a pilot study to increase screening for domestic abuse show markedly inconsistent results depending on when and by whom the screening was carried out, what is the first factor to consider?

a. Population
b. Timing
c. Location
d. Training

86. Which of the following is a valid source of information about evidence-based public health approaches?

a. AHRQ Innovations Exchange
b. WebMD
c. Centers for Medicare and Medicaid (CMS)
d. Medline Plus

87. When sending an email to communicate with a priority population, the health education specialist should be aware that the primary determinant in whether the person reads the email or not is often the

a. content of the email.
b. sender.
c. subject line.
d. time email is sent.

88. The health education specialist has located a data collection instrument that appears to be well-constructed and sensitive for the desired measures. However, the readability level is far too high for the priority population, which has low literacy rates, so the instrument would have to be substantially rewritten. The health education specialist's first response should be to

  a. attempt to locate a different instrument.
  b. rewrite the text of the instrument to simplify the content.
  c. use only the parts of the instrument that have lower readability levels.
  d. construct an instrument that is appropriate.

89. If the health education specialist would like to utilize smart phones to communicate with and send information to members of a priority population, the first step should be to

  a. provide smart phones to the priority population.
  b. survey the population regarding smart phone use.
  c. advise the participants that they need to get smart phones.
  d. apply for a grant to help participants pay for smart phones.

90. A health education specialist works for a large industrial corporation and is selecting technology to manage program data for a health initiative. The first step should be to

  a. choose an operating system.
  b. gather information about available technology.
  c. determine the funds available for purchasing technology.
  d. assess existing technology and resources.

91. The most important factor in ensuring consistency in implementation of a health education program is usually

  a. size of program.
  b. priority population.
  c. supervision.
  d. training.

92. The health education specialist has developed an instructional computer lab as part of an educational program but has had reports that staff members are monopolizing the computers and using them for personal projects and business despite staff being told that the computers are to be used only by program participants. If the health education specialist plans to monitor computer use, the first step is to

  a. install monitoring software.
  b. provide a written policy.
  c. warn staff members.
  d. consult an attorney.

93. The health education specialist is concerned about the misuse of alcohol and medications among older adults in the community and plans a program to assess needs, identify resources, and educate staff and older adults about the dangers of misuse and programs to assist in more responsible use. When conducting a survey as part of a needs assessment, which type of survey is likely to have the lowest response rate?

    a. Mail
    b. Email
    c. Telephone
    d. One-on-one

94. The health education specialist is concerned about the misuse of alcohol and medications among older adults in the community and plans a program to assess needs, identify resources, and educate staff and older adults about the dangers of misuse and programs to assist in more responsible use. The health education specialist wants to establish a resource database that includes resources that may aid in the development of the program and provide ongoing support. The first step should be to

    a. begin making telephone calls.
    b. review a directory of agencies and organizations.
    c. determine the types of resources needed.
    d. ask advice of key informants in the community.

95. The health education specialist is concerned about the misuse of alcohol and medications among older adults in the community and plans a program to assess needs, identify resources, and educate staff and older adults about the dangers of misuse and programs to assist in more responsible use. The health education specialist plans to present workshops at senior citizen's centers and retirement homes about the signs of alcohol and medication misuse. Part of the presentation includes a 20-minute video, which will be preceded by an introduction of the main points of the video. What is the most valuable use of time following the video?

    a. Have a discussion period.
    b. Take a break.
    c. Conduct a survey.
    d. Dismiss the group.

96. The health education specialist is concerned about the misuse of alcohol and medications among older adults in the community and plans a program to assess needs, identify resources, and educate staff and older adults about the dangers of misuse and programs to assist in more responsible use. An older adult in attendance asks about an article about medication misuse in the popular press, wondering if the information is valid. The article summarizes a study done by a university and discusses its ramifications. Regarding the validity of the information, the health education specialist should

    a. reassure the individual that the information is valid.
    b. offer to research the primary source of information about the study.
    c. tell the individual that the information is not valid.
    d. advise the individual that there's no way to know if the information is valid.

97. While developing a plan to increase prenatal care among a priority population of non-Spanish-speaking indigenous Mayan immigrants from Guatemala, the health education specialist has been unable to find appropriate materials and has, therefore, developed handouts, checklists, and guides independently with the help of a professional translator. Before full implementation, the health education specialist should

    a. ask a second translator to evaluate materials.
    b. try again to find materials for this population.
    c. ask key community members to evaluate the materials.
    d. pilot test the materials.

98. The health education specialist has convinced the school to place only healthy snacks in the vending machines when implementing a program to improve student nutrition and reduce obesity, but the result has been a sharp decline in purchases from the vending machines because the students are unhappy with the choices. This is an example of

    a. reciprocal determinism.
    b. collective efficacy.
    c. self-regulation.
    d. emotional coping response.

99. An example of a *tailored message* is a(n)

    a. message that has been modified to reflect literacy level of recipient.
    b. message emailed to a priority population based on shared interests.
    c. message sent in response to request for information.
    d. Internet pop-up ad with health information based on the individual's Internet searches.

100. If the health education specialist has placed information about self-breast exam on a website and wants to determine if information has been viewed by an adequate number of people, the best method is to

    a. observe for increases in the number of mammograms.
    b. use a web counter to track traffic to the website.
    c. ask viewers to complete a survey.
    d. ask local practitioners to survey patients.

101. As part of a program to decrease violence in the schools, the health education specialist has been educating staff and students about the use of messaging and other social media to intimidate, threaten, and damage the reputation of students and faculty. This type of behavior is classified as

    a. violence.
    b. bullying.
    c. electronic aggression.
    d. assault.

102. As a member of the curriculum committee in a school district, the health education specialist helps to select health topics and instructional materials. The health education specialist has received dozens of books, pamphlets, videos, and other materials from publishers and government agencies to review. The first step should be to

a. separate the material into categories.
b. review costs of materials.
c. for a sub-committee to assist.
d. develop/find a materials review form.

103. When enrolling patients in a heart healthy program to help them better control their blood pressure and cholesterol levels through diet, exercise, and lifestyle changes, the first action should be to

a. teach self-monitoring of VS.
b. discuss dietary modifications.
c. define lifestyle changes.
d. gather baseline data.

104. As the date for implementation of a new program nears, the health education specialist finds that one important component of the project has lagged behind and cannot be fully completed by the target date. The best solution is to

a. delay implementation.
b. proceed with full implementation.
c. replace staff working on the component.
d. carry out a partial implementation.

105. Which of the following is a limitation of the lecture format for teaching a group of participants in a health education program?

a. Serving multiple patients in a short time
b. Delivering exactly the same information to all of group members
c. Supplementing the lecture with audiovisual materials
d. Having shared interests among group members

106. When assessing readiness for implementation of an organization's health promotion plan for a priority population comprised primarily of Chinese Americans, the health education specialist should focus on

a. interest in the program.
b. Chinese cultural traditions.
c. allies in the community.
d. available resources and leadership commitment.

107. When utilizing direct mailing as part of a marketing plan, the best method is likely

a. targeted mailing.
b. mass mailing.
c. mailing by request.
d. mailing to key informants.

108. When implementing a worksite health promotion effort that includes hiring and managing personnel, the best way to avoid conflict in the workplace is by

    a. tying salary to performance.
    b. hiring personnel recommended by coworkers.
    c. clearly outlining expectations.
    d. clearly outlining disciplinary actions.

109. When applying the Theory of Planned Behavior in a program to decrease smoking among adolescents, the health education specialist recruits coaches, teachers, and student leaders that the adolescents respect to encourage the smokers to stop smoking. This is an example of utilizing the construct of

    a. behavioral beliefs.
    b. attitude toward the behavior.
    c. control beliefs.
    d. subjective norm.

110. The health education specialist wants to use social modeling according to concepts of Social Cognitive Theory (SCT) to influence students at a university to develop strategies to avoid situations in which date rape may occur. An example of social modeling is having

    a. peers to talk about strategies.
    b. famous people to talk about strategies.
    c. social gatherings to promote awareness.
    d. data to show the rates of date rape.

111. The health education specialist has recommended that clinicians use the Rapid Estimate of Adult Literacy in Medicine (REALM) instrument to assess health literacy with patients in response to a number of incidents in which patients did not understand directions regarding medication use. This test requires the patients to

    a. carry out a self-assessment regarding medical terms.
    b. answer a number of questions about health-related issues.
    c. read a list of medical words and lay terms for body parts and disorders.
    d. read a passage about a medical topic and explain the contents.

112. If utilizing the Health Belief Model as the basis for a communication strategy to increase participation in smoking cessation programs, the health education specialist must survey to find

    a. the number of smokers.
    b. the average age of smokers.
    c. perceptions about smoking.
    d. people with smoking-associated disorders.

113. Key informants of a priority population are usually

    a. the oldest members of the population.
    b. those in positions of power or influence.
    c. those who are not in positions of power.
    d. younger members of the population.

114. When assessing learning domains, which domain should be assessed first if the person must learn skills, such as monitoring diabetes and injecting insulin?

a. Affective
b. Cognitive
c. Psychomotor
d. Order doesn't matter

115. A health education specialist who understands the importance of building relationships with many individuals in a priority population and encouraging people to work together is interested in investing in

a. cultural capital.
b. economic capital.
c. social capital.
d. environmental capital.

116. Which of the following is not a true statement about the use of focus groups in the development of a needs assessment survey?

a. A focus group is a good way to obtain information and identify issues, concerns, or strengths by posing specific questions to be discussed using a small group of people
b. A focus group should consist of a mixed group of people in order to get a variety of opinions concerning specific questions to be discussed
c. The facilitator of the focus group should try to keep the conversation on topic by gently veering back to the question at hand but should try to let the participants speak freely
d. After the focus group is finished, the information should be compiled based on the answers to the questions and categorized within each question

117. When collecting health-related data, sources of secondary data include all of the following except:

a. Observation
b. Vital records
c. Peer-reviewed journals
d. United States Census Bureau

118. When identifying factors that influence health, addressing which of the following factors would be least likely to make a large impact on the overall health of a community?

a. Lifestyle factors such as smoking
b. Environmental factors such as access to affordable food
c. Psychosocial factors such as social supports
d. Biological factors such as genetics

119. What is the final step in the needs assessment process?

a. Validating the needs that have been identified
b. Identifying gaps in healthcare services
c. Data analysis
d. Conduct a resource inventory

120. Which of the following would be the most expensive survey method to use for data collection?

a. Telephone
b. Mail
c. Face-to-face
d. Internet

121. What is the name of the term that measures an outcome that is designed to identify the rate of occurrence of an issue?

a. Validation
b. Clinical indicator
c. Pretest
d. Resource inventory

122. Once a specific population has been identified through the needs assessment for health education, what would be one of the next steps in the planning process?

a. Approach local leaders and community groups to obtain support for the project
b. Begin to advertise the program to the specific population the program will be targeted toward
c. Develop learning objectives
d. Identify educational strategies that will be used such as workshops or seminars

123. Which of the following would be the least effective goal of a program in an area where the rate of low-birth-weight infants is elevated?

a. Reduce the number of births to teenage mothers
b. Increase access to family planning services to Caucasian women between the ages of 18 and 35
c. Reduce the rate of smoking among pregnant women
d. Reduce the rate of unplanned pregnancies among women who are eligible for Medicaid

124. When planning a health education program, it important to remember that not all participants will want to learn. What would be the most effective way to help maximize learning?

a. Provide materials that the participant can read
b. Quickly move through the material, covering each topic one time
c. Have the presenter stand in front of the group and lecture
d. Use audiovisual aids such as PowerPoint during the presentation, and allow time for discussion

125. In the PRECEDE-PROCEED model, what step should be taken in phase 5?

a. Epidemiological assessment
b. Administrative and policy assessment
c. Ecological assessment
d. Social assessment

126. What is the name of the planning model that utilizes five phases (goals selection, intervention planning, program development, implementation preparations, and evaluation)?

a. CDCynergy
b. PRECEDE-PROCEED
c. MATCH
d. Social marketing

127. Which of the following would be an example of a learning objective?

a. Participants will be able to reduce total fat intake by 25% by the end of the nutrition program
b. Within six months, 50% of participants will have lowered their total serum cholesterol by at least 30 points
c. Participants will reduce the risk factors for heart disease
d. The participant will be able to identify three sources of saturated fat in the diet

128. The statement "The city will have a 10% reduction in the number of days with poor air quality" is an example of:

a. Environmental objective
b. Ecological objective
c. Behavioral objective
d. Administrative objective

129. Obesity has been identified during a needs assessment in a rural area where there is a high percentage of families that use food stamp benefits. Which of the following would not be the most effective component of the health education plan in terms of implementation?

a. Organize a community weight loss competition with monetary incentives, such as gift cards to local grocery stores
b. Provide free seminars in supermarkets to teach residents how to plan healthful meals on a budget
c. Work with the school to encourage a healthy exercise competition by rewarding the classroom with the most minutes of exercise in a given period with a special prize
d. Encourage residents to join the local health club

130. Developing a community garden in a local park would be most effective in what setting?

a. University
b. Health clinic
c. Town
d. Place of business

131. All of the following are benefits of a pretest except:

a. To be able to assess knowledge of the intervention group prior to initiating health education
b. To initiate behavior changes prior to starting the health education program
c. To determine what the strengths and weaknesses are of the intervention group
d. To determine the level of comprehension prior to starting health education

132. Which of the following would be the best example of cultural competence in the workplace?

a. Develop a zero-tolerance policy for discrimination based on ethnic, religious, gender, or sexual orientation identify
b. Hire bilingual staff to assist in education
c. Plan cultural diversity workshops
d. Assess individual values and beliefs toward various ethnic or religious groups that are part of the workplace

133. Which of the following is not a valid statement in relation to instructional technology and health education?

a. Using various search engines to find information is simple to do and does not require specialized knowledge
b. A working knowledge of PowerPoint, word processing, and spreadsheet software is important
c. Email remains an important tool for communication
d. A health educator must be familiar with various forms of social media, such as Facebook and Twitter, in order to be effective

134. What is the first phase that occurs during the implementation of a health education program?

a. Resource estimation
b. Gain acceptance of the program
c. Program management
d. Sustaining a program

135. What is the name of the term used to describe when all facets of the health program are introduced simultaneously?

a. Pilot phase
b. Field testing
c. Immersion implementation
d. Total implementation

136. What is the name of the model or theory used in education that deals with the stages of change?

a. Transtheoretical model
b. Health belief model
c. Social cognitive theory
d. Diffusion of innovations theory

137. A 45-year-old male has been smoking for 25 years. He understands the dangers of smoking and has tried many times in the past to quit. He has picked a quit date that is three weeks from now and has made an appointment the next week with his physician to discuss starting a nicotine replacement therapy program. What stage of change is this man currently in?

a. Precontemplation
b. Termination
c. Preparation
d. Maintenance

138. What is the name of the legal term that is used to explain the risks and benefits of a program or treatment?

a. HIPAA
b. Risk management
c. Durable power of attorney
d. Informed consent

139. A medium-sized company in the private sector is introducing a wellness program aimed at reducing cholesterol levels and blood pressure. What would be a good way to promote participation in this program?

a. Require all employees to have a mandatory physical for baseline readings with their primary care physician, then require follow up every three months
b. Offer mobile cholesterol and blood pressure screenings and follow-ups as well as gift cards for participation
c. Request all employees to complete a health risk assessment to determine possible participants
d. Send out a wellness newsletter that outlines ways to reduce both blood pressure and cholesterol for those who are interested

140. Which of the following would not be a recommended strategy for effectively teaching a health education curriculum to students of middle-school age?

a. Tries to address the topic being presented by relating it to social factors, values, and skills of the group
b. Addresses perceptions related to the risks or benefits of a certain behavior
c. Tries to increase student knowledge of the topic by utilizing scientific facts and theories
d. Incorporates ways to avoid or address risky situations related to the topic that may confront the students

141. What is the approximate average attention span for listening to a lecture without interruptions and being able to maintain focus?

a. 10 to 12 minutes
b. 12 to 20 minutes
c. 20 to 26 minutes
d. 24 to 35 minutes

142. You are doing Internet research for an upcoming health education program. By looking at a URL, you would be able to determine all of the following except:

a. If the Web site is an individual's personal page
b. What type of domain the Web site originates from
c. Who the publisher of the page is
d. If the information has been verified as safe

143. What type of research study design is considered the gold standard?

a. Observational
b. Cohort
c. Randomized controlled
d. Meta-analysis

144. A person that is involved in a research study is protected by which of the following?

a. NIH
b. EPA
c. USDA
d. IRB

145. Which of the following would not be a term used in descriptive statistics?

a. Measures of quantitative analysis
b. Measures of dispersion
c. Measures of kurtosis
d. Measures of skew

146. Measures of central tendency would include all of the following terms EXCEPT:

a. Mode
b. Intermediate
c. Mean
d. Median

147. Which of the following statements is most accurate about the development of a data measurement instrument?

a. Developing a new data measurement instrument is an easy process
b. Many data collection instruments are copyrighted, but the authors are often willing to share with other researchers
c. Most authors are happy to share their data collection instruments with anyone who asks
d. It is a relatively simple process to find an established data collection instrument

148. What is the first question that must be answered when embarking on a strategic planning process?

a. Where do we want to go?
b. What path do we take to get there?
c. Where are we now?
d. What is our time frame for achieving our goals?

149. What is the most effective method of recruiting volunteers to assist with health education programs?

a. Media campaign
b. Posting on a bulletin board in a highly visible area
c. Identifying individuals who attend other community programs
d. By personally inviting an individual

150. Which of the following would be least helpful in the training of volunteers?

a. Introduce the volunteer to the organization and the staff
b. Provide a mandatory training day offered once per month before service can begin
c. Describe the mission and structure of the organization
d. Take the time to get to know individual volunteers to find out what their goals and concerns are about their service commitment

151. When interviewing a potential volunteer, the candidate asks about expenses and reimbursement. What document would most likely address this?

a. Confidentiality agreement
b. Volunteer application form
c. Volunteer policies and procedures
d. Performance review

152. What type of information should not be used for screening potential volunteers?

a. Medical history
b. Criminal background check
c. Driving records
d. Personal references

153. When developing health education materials, what is one of the most important guidelines?

a. Use bright colors
b. Use plain language
c. Use a large font
d. Have the materials translated into other languages

154. If you are trying to research osteoporosis, which database would be least appropriate to use?

a. PubMed
b. Medline
c. Cochrane Review
d. ERIC

155. As part of your responsibilities as a health education specialist, you need to evaluate Web sites before passing the information along to your program participants. Which of the following is the best Web site that you can utilize to find other reliable health-related Web sites?

a. www.webmd.com
b. www.kidshealth.org
c. www.healthfinder.gov
d. www.health.com

156. What is the main difference between an internal consultant and an external consultant?

a. An internal consultant provides more technical assistance
b. An external consultant requires more specialized knowledge than an internal consultant
c. A contract is usually required for the services of an external consultant but not for an internal consultant
d. An internal consultant performs tasks that are more process oriented

157. A task force is being established to address underage drinking in a community that has experienced a large number of incidents involving minors. Which of the following groups would be most important to include in order to make the greatest possible impact?

a. High school students
b. Teachers
c. Law enforcement
d. Youth pastors

158. A program being developed to address smoking would be least effective in which of the following populations?

a. Individuals who live in the Midwest
b. Individuals of American-Indian/Alaska-native/African-American descent
c. Individuals with an income level at or slightly above the poverty level
d. Individuals with a college education

159. When serving as a health education consultant, which of the following would be an appropriate document to follow to ensure ethical behavior and decision-making?

a. Code of Ethics for the Health Education Profession
b. HIPAA
c. FERPA
d. The organization's policy and procedure manual

160. All of the following are new topics for Healthy People 2020 EXCEPT:

a. Global health
b. Adolescent health
c. Health communication and health information technology
d. Healthcare-associated infections

161. A health educator has developed a comprehensive contact list that includes a variety of other health professionals working in various jobs in related to health. The health educator will use this list to select another professional if assistance is needed with an issue or if he or she wants an opinion on something. For example, if the health educator has questions about diet or nutrition, he or she may call a registered dietitian that works at the local hospital. This is called:

a. Consulting
b. Networking
c. Liaison
d. Resource

162. In a community setting, other names for a lay health education specialist would include all of the following EXCEPT:

a. CHES
b. Promotores de salud
c. Community health advisor
d. Community health advocate

163. Which of the following is a true statement about areas where there is a high rate of low literacy skills?

a. Five percent of all adults are not literate, and the areas impacted in the United States are located mainly in the South
b. Most healthcare providers assess each individual to ensure average literacy when beginning any type of health education
c. Populations with low literacy skills are able to understand their medical conditions through the use of the Internet
d. Populations with low literacy skills tend to have poorer health and higher healthcare costs

164. A health education specialist needs to contact her state representative to provide input on a proposed health legislation. What is the least effective way to contact the legislator?

a. Form letter sent through the U.S. Postal Service
b. Email
c. Telephone
d. A faxed handwritten note

165. A health education specialist must develop a plan for professional growth. This may include all of the following EXCEPT:

a. Attend professional meetings to network and stay current
b. Stay up to date on technology skills including PowerPoint, Internet search, social media, and developing Web pages
c. Obtaining 100 hours of continuing education contact hours every 5 years to maintain certification
d. Obtaining a master's degree in an appropriate area such as master's of education

Answers and Explanations

1. B: Quarantining of children infected with measles is an example of a secondary intervention aimed at preventing communicable disease in a priority population. Interventions:

Primary: Those interventions intended to prevent the disease from occurring in the first place, such as by chlorinating water or carrying out immunization programs.

Secondary: Those interventions utilized after the disease has occurred with the aim to prevent the condition from worsening or spreading, such as by quarantining children infected with measles.

Tertiary: Those interventions to reduce or alleviate the impact of disease, such as post-meningitis rehabilitation programs.

2. A: If a staff member in a health education program to increase HIV/AIDS testing and safe sex practices among gay males in an inner city posted personal information about one client on a social media site, this is a violation of the ethical principle of confidentiality. Because the program is health-related, this is also a violation of HIPAA regulations. Even though the person was not named, personal information may make identification of the person possible.

3. C: If the health education specialist is planning a class exercise in which the class members will need to work in small groups, the best room seating arrangement is probably cluster seating in which four chairs are placed together around a center point. This facilitates working in groups and collaborating and is especially valuable when students are learning from each other and participating in hands-on learning. However, the chair positions mean that some members will have their backs to the front of the room and may need to move their chairs to face the instructor.

4. D: If the health education specialist is engaged in a campaign to encourage employees at a large company to have flu shots as one method to decrease seasonal absenteeism, the best strategy for gaining attention about the issue is probably paycheck stuffers because people are less likely to ignore notices presented with their paychecks than other types of marketing. Another method to encourage flu shots is to offer them at the worksite during work hours and/or to offer incentives.

5. B: If the health education specialist wants visual data to show health care trends regarding healthcare quality and disparities in order to justify a program, the best source is probably AHRQ, which has compiled annual statistics about healthcare quality and statistics for over a decade. AHRQ provides a number of different data sources, including the Medical Expenditure Panel Survey and the Healthcare Cost and Utilization Project, as well as evidence-based reports.

6. C: When the health education specialist explains why technology resources benefit the priority population, the health education specialist is applying the ethical principle of beneficence. Beneficence requires a focus on the needs of the priority population and the aim to intervene for a positive purpose. Justice involves equal distribution of resources although this may vary according to need. Veracity is being open and truthful while nonmaleficence is avoiding harm to others and is closely allied to beneficence.

7. B: If the health education specialist is implementing a diabetic clinic as part of a health education program to decrease rates of diabetes and diabetic complications among a priority population comprised primarily of undocumented Mexican immigrants with no insurance, but only a few people have used the clinic because of fears about deportation, the best marketing plan is probably

129

gaining support of key informants in the community. These must be people that the population trusts and may include community leaders, priests or other spiritual advisors, and employers.

8. A: In order to assess progress in achieving objectives, the health education specialist must first determine indicators—that which will be measured. Indicators should be identified as part of the planning process so that when the program is implemented there is a clear understanding of what will be measured to determine if objectives are met and when and how the measurements will take place. When possible, measures should provide quantitative data although qualitative data may be equally valuable.

9. C: Utilizing the social analysis network tool PARTNER (Program to Analyze, Record, and Track Networks to Enhance Relationship) to monitor a partnership allows the health education specialist to (1) create visuals showing connections, (2) assess network scores, and (3) assess outcomes measures:

Create visuals: Showing connections and relationships.

Assess Network scores: Measures regarding relationships, trusts, and values.

Assess outcomes measures: Showing achievements.

10. A: If the health education specialist working for a nonprofit healthcare organization needs to present the results of data collection to the board of directors of the organization, the best way to present the information is through charts that provide visual representations of the data and raw data. Because the board of directors oversees the organization, the members should have access to all data. However, the data should be summarized as well so that it is more easily accessible.

11. D: When applying Bridge's Transition Model to help people in an organization cope with change in the initial stage when they are uncomfortable and/or resistant to change (ending, losing, letting go), the health education specialist should listen to people, allowing them to freely express opinions, and communicate openly, impressing on people the positive aspects of change and their roles in the change. In stage 2 (neutral zone), confusion and uncertainly are common, so the health education specialist should provide support and guidance. The last stage (new beginning) when people begin to accept changes, the health education specialist should celebrate change, reward people, and commit to change.

12. B: If members of a priority population take exercise classes and participate in smoking cessation programs, the need for these services would be classified as expressed because they can be observed. Actual needs are those that are inferred by comparing like areas or populations, such as the lack of recreational facilities. Normative needs indicate a discrepancy between the status of one population and another. Perceived needs are those a population believes are necessary.

13. A: The first step in the marketing process is to analyze the situation. The health education specialist needs a good overview. As part of this step, the problems and population affected should be identified and current behaviors and replacement behaviors analyzed. The environment in which changes will occur must be carefully assessed and then all possible solutions outlined. Step 2 is to select the most appropriate approaches and determine marketing's role. Step 3 is to select goals and objectives and step 4 to segment/select the propriety populations.

14. C: If the health education specialist has developed a new protocol and tools for teaching new parents to properly care for infants, before implementing the program, the health education specialist should carry out pilot testing to determine if the protocol and tools work well or need to be modified. Pilot testing can help to identify strengths of the program as well as problems and to determine if training and materials provide adequate preparation for staff.

15. B: If the health education specialist has received notice from a community foundation that, because of an increase in funding for another agency and decreased revenue, an anticipated grant cannot be provided to implement the program the health education specialist has developed, the first step in dealing with this barrier to implementation should be to search for alternative funding sources. Developing a program without first securing funding is never prudent. If other funding sources cannot be identified, then the program may need to be delayed, modified, or cancelled.

16. D: When utilizing data mining as part of data collection, data mining is used primarily for predictive analysis. For example, data mining of hospital admission and readmission data may provide information that allows the health education specialist to predict the patients that are most likely to be readmitted to the hospital because of noncompliance with treatment. The health education specialist can then target interventions for this priority population in order to improve compliance and reduce readmissions.

17. A: When using the Ecological Systems Model to assess the capacity of stakeholders to meet program goals, the health education specialist should recognize that multiple factors affect behavior. Ecology refers to the interrelationship between an individual and the environment about that individual. The ecological factors may be intrapersonal, interpersonal, community, organizational, environmental, or policy-associated. These influences interact in multiple ways that may not be predictable, so many issues must be considered during assessment: Do stakeholders have the time, the resources, the motivation, the support, the need, and the ability?

18. C: While publicly criticizing the community for inaction regarding a free clinic to serve the homeless population as well as undocumented immigrants may, in fact, catch the attention of some people, generally speaking it is better to use a positive approach when trying to engage stakeholders rather than a negative approach. The health education specialist should focus on benefits to the community and should identify available resources, allies (including other groups or organizations with similar interests), and adversaries.

19. D: If a community needs assessment shows markedly increased rates of HIV among injection drug users, an example of an appropriate outcome based on this assessment is establishment of a needle exchange program because needle sharing is a common means of transmission of HIV. This outcome directly applies to the need. Outcomes that call for the "elimination" of something are usually unrealistic. Increased punishment for drug dealers does not address the problem of HIV infection.

20. B: If the health education specialist commits the public health department to work with another community agency to promote the common goal of reducing HIV infections related to injection drug use, the type of intervention the health education specialist is utilizing is collaboration. Collaboration involves two or more individuals or organizations working together to meet a common goal in such a way that the sum of the whole is greater than the sum of the parts.

21. B: The most likely impact of a strictly enforced local ordinance against sleeping on the streets or in the parks overnight in the downtown area in order to remove the homeless is a shift of the homeless population to outside of the downtown area. Ideally, there would be an increase in shelters, but this, unfortunately, is rarely the case as such ordinances are usually intended to rid the area of the homeless rather than to accommodate them.

22. C: There are a number of different types of non-governmental health agencies:

Voluntary health agencies: Including the American Heart Association and American Cancer Society

Philanthropic foundations: Including the Ford Foundation and Rockefeller Foundation.

Fraternal, religious, and service organizations: Including Shriner's, Salvation Army, Lion's, and Catholic Relief Fund.

Professional health associations: Including The American Academy of Health Behavior and American Alliance for Health, Physical Education, Recreation, and Dance.

23. D: When storing and utilizing large amounts of personal data about members of a priority population, the primary concern is security. Access to the data should be carefully controlled through passwords or other forms of identification. Personally identifiable information (PII), which includes any information that can be utilized to identify, locate, or contact a person (such as name, address, email address, telephone number, fingerprints, photographic image, and Social Security number), must be secured and confidentiality assured.

24. A: The step in media literacy that the health education specialist is utilizing when using media devices to convene a priority population is reaction, the last step in the 4-step process. The first step, awareness, involves exploration of media sources through accessing information from a variety of different sources. The second step involves analysis of the various messages by comparing and contrasting. The third step involves reflection to evaluate the implicit and explicit messages from the individual's perception.

25. C: When considering the best method of surveying a population for a needs assessment, the first thing to consider is the characteristics of the target population. The health education specialist must consider such factors as age, ethnic background, and socioeconomic status in order to pick a survey method that is likely to receive the best return. As preparation for more formal surveys, the health education specialist may conduct a literature review and windshield assessments.

26. B: If the health education specialist plans to conduct community forums and to interview key informants regarding the needs of a priority population for health-related information, prior to the forums and interviews, the health education specialist should review literature and social indicators, such as census data, health statistical data, and welfare data so that the health education specialist comes armed with some information. The health education specialist may also carry out a windshield assessment to get an overall impression of the community.

27. C: If a television ad for a health campaign has a large reach (the number of people who were exposed to or viewed the ad) and a poor recall (number of people who recalled seeing the ad or remembered the message), then the problem is probably the presentation of the message. Television ads are brief—usually 15, 30, or 60 seconds. Thirty-second ads usually show better return on investment than 15-second ads. Ads must rapidly catch the viewers' attention and be memorable enough to ensure recall.

28. B: If the health education specialist is concerned about healthcare disparities, the heath education specialist's advocacy efforts should begin with personal practice, ensuring equity in provision of care and selection of the priority population. When developing programs, the health care specialist should consider those in the community who lack adequate care, such as immigrants, people with low incomes, and the homeless. Other advocacy efforts may include joining local, state, and national organizations to actively lobby to overcome health disparities.

29. A: If the health education specialist has placed information about the need for vaccinations on a kiosk in a local mall, the type of communication channel the health education specialist utilizing is the community channel. Community channels also include school campaigns, town hall meetings, community events, faith-based campaigns, community educational programs, public speeches. Community channels often engender trust because they may be familiar and may reach a large audience; however, community channels may be difficult to establish and behavior change resulting from community channels is difficult to measure.

30. D: When prioritizing community needs for preventive efforts, the three primary considerations are:

- Leading causes of death/morbidity: This information available from the National Center for Health Statistics and usually includes such disorders as heart disease, cancer, stroke, and COPD.
- Years of potential life lost: These include disorders that are life threatening or may shorten life, such as diabetes and cancer.
- Economic costs: These costs are usually to society as a whole, but they may be focused more locally, such as costs to a city.

31. A: Based on the information in the graph, the two factors that are most critical in determining exposure to second-hand smoke are the poverty level and race. Home ownership is closely aligned with the poverty level because those below the poverty level are often unable to own a home, and exposure to secondhand smoke is higher among those below the poverty level. Of the three ethnic groups, Blacks have exposure to secondhand smoke at more than double the rates of whites or Mexican-Americans.

32. D: When conducting a culture audit of an organization, the finding that would be cause for most concern is if the organization employees were afraid to give their opinions. People who are afraid of repercussions if they speak up are unlikely to be creative in problem solving or motivated to improve an organization. Employees can be committed to an organization even if they believe their salaries are low if they feel that they are otherwise treated well. In most organization, key decision-makers are readily identified, and differences of opinion about vision and mission are common.

33. C: According to Kotter's 8-step change model, the health education specialist should convince at least 75% of key staff that organizational change is warranted. This is part of the first step, which is to establish a sense of urgency for change. Step two is to form a coalition, step 3 to create a vision, step four to communicate the vision however possible, step five to empower others, step 6 to plan visible performance improvements, step 7 to consolidate improvements to increase credibility and facilitate more change, and finally step 8, which is to institutionalize the changes.

34. A: If a public health organization is utilizing the Six Sigma model for program improvement, the health education specialist should expect much emphasis to be placed on data collection as the model is data-driven. The goal of Six Sigma is to eliminate "defects" in processes. The perception of the customer is a key element because the customer defines elements that are "critical to quality" (CTQ). Six Sigma includes two types of improvement programs: DMAIC (define, measure, analyze, improve, control) for existing processes that require improvement and DMADV (define, measure, analyze, design, verify) for development of new processes.

35. B: When conveying health information to a consumer, it is critically important to consider not only the message but also the type of consumer. In this case, the primary focus of the presentation about the HPV vaccination should probably be on preventing cervical and penile cancer because of the conservative nature of the population and their concerns about promiscuity. Cancer is less emotionally charged as a topic than sexually transmitted diseases, and this focus on cancer targets a common fear.

36. C: Starting a petition is support of an initiative to increase funding for homeless shelters is an example of grassroots lobbying, an advocacy strategy. Holding town hall meetings is another example. Other strategies include registering to vote and participating in a voter registration drive; contributing to legislative allies; contacting policymakers directly in person, by phone, or by email; using the Internet to spread information; carrying out media advocacy; and using social media to influence others.

37. D: If the health education specialist has developed a Facebook page and Twitter account in order to use social media to reach people in the community and has approximately 3500 followers, the health education specialist should plan on updating the Facebook page with new information one to five times per month. Studies show that making more frequent updates doesn't affect traffic until the followers exceed 60,000. Too frequent updates of information often result in updates with little actual content. It's better to update less frequently but with valuable information for the consumer.

38. C: If a coalition of community agencies has come together to develop a plan to promote reduction in obesity through healthier lifestyle choices, the next step should be to elicit community input regarding the plan. The health education specialist should seek key representatives in the priority population as well as key individuals in the organizations. Surveys may be carried out and community meetings held in easily accessible locations in order to encourage participation.

39. A: While all of these are important criteria for volunteers, the most important is usually the skills the person has. Before recruiting volunteers, the health education specialist should outline the tasks that the volunteers will perform and consider how important they are to the implementation process. While it may be tempting to accept all volunteers, carefully screening them to find those who are most capable is often a better strategy.

40. B: In a needs assessment, *capacity* refers to assets or resources that can be utilized to improve health or empower a population. Capacity can include skills, groups, individuals, and resources, such as equipment, facilities, and finances. A needs assessment should assess capacity, including gaps in capacity that may require strengthening or may negatively impact a program. Latent capacity, resources that are available but not utilized or recognized, should also be identified as part of assessment.

41. D: An organization's mission statement should include the organization's purpose, showing why the organization exists and describing, in broad terms, the functions of the organizations. Mission statements are usually one sentence in length although a short narrative may be used as well. The mission statement should be considered a long-term overriding purpose that may be achieved in various ways. A vision statement, on the other hand, should show the desired outcomes of a program.

42. A: If a community needs assessment is based on results of an Internet survey only, the ethical principle that may be violated is *equity* because those without access to the Internet will not be represented in the survey. Additionally, some age groups, particularly young adults, are more likely to respond to Internet surveys than others, such as older adults, who may feel less comfortable with or less trusting of electronic media and the Internet.

43. D: According to the graph, the group that showed an increase in motor vehicle-related deaths between 2009 and 2010 is females 20 to 24 years although the increase is quite small. All other groups showed a decline in deaths over that same period. Interestingly, while females have an overall lower rate of motor vehicle deaths than males, the overall change in rates from 2000 to 2010 declined less markedly for females than males, declining only about 5 to 10%.

44. A: Based on the information in the graph, the group that would most benefit from a targeted education program regarding motor vehicle safety is males 20 to 24 years because their overall rate, while showing a marked decline after 2007 is still the highest with the rate dropping from about 42% to about 28% in 2010. Males 15 to 19 years have rates that declined from about 34% to 18% in 2010. These rates are both higher than females who ranged from 15% to 18% in 2000 to around 10% in 2010.

45. B: The National Task Force on the Preparation and Practice of Health Educators was first established in 1978, representing the official beginning of the certification process recognizing the profession of health education. However, the first CHES exam was not administered until 1990 and the Code of Ethics for Health Education Profession adopted until 2000. The CHES certification program was accredited by the NCCA in 2008. Over time, the professional title changed from "health educator" to "health education specialist."

46. C: If searching for statistics regarding rates of tuberculosis, an appropriate source of secondary data is the CDC. The CDCs National Center for Health Statistics provides statistics about a wide range of diseases, injuries, life stages, populations, health care, and insurance. The CDC provides state, regional, and national data from both required and voluntary reporting. Data is available free of charge from the CDC and most is available on the Internet and can be downloaded.

47. B: If two organizations have agreed to collaborate on an educational program as separate entities with no sharing of financial resources and each organization carrying out different functions, the organizations should likely have a memorandum of understanding (MOU), which outlines the different functions and expectations. An MOU is less formal than a contract and more formal than a verbal agreement although it is often considered legally binding, depending on the wording used in the agreement.

48. A: If utilizing a logic model to show how a program aligns with the mission and goals of an organization, the health education specialist would typically develops a flowchart with at least three categories: input, output, and outcomes. A logic model often begins with a problem statement and goal. Inputs may include such things as resources, rationales, assumptions, interventions, and participation. Outputs are completed activities, and outcomes are classified into three categories: short-term, intermediate, and long-term.

49. B: If the health education specialist is assessing the potential use of the smart watch, such as the Apple Watch, and software applications to remotely monitor the vital signs and exercise of participants in a health improvement program, the primary concern about using this new technology is likely cost. While the technology may be ideal for the intended purpose, when program participants need equipment that costs hundreds of dollars and is not yet widely used, then this poses the ethical problem of equity.

50. C: If the health education specialist plans to present the rationale for a community program to a coalition of community agencies and organizations that meet monthly, the best method of communication is probably an oral presentation at the monthly meeting. This gives the health education specialist the opportunity to meet with key members and to answer questions. A written report should also be presented so that the members of the coalition can take it with them for further review.

51. A: Because the county is widespread with a large city, suburbs, towns and rural areas, probably the best method of implementation is phased-in implementation by location. For example, the program may begin in one small town or one section of the city and then after a specified period of time (one month for example) another area is added. Full implementation of the program may put too much burden on existing staff and require a considerable expenditure of resources.

52. A: If a health education specialist working for a large business wants to develop a multi-faceted fitness program for employees but must secure resources through a request to top management, when preparing the presentation, the health education specialist should focus on benefits to the business—such as more motivated staff, decreased injuries, and decreased utilization of sick time. Business management is often most concerned with return on investment, so the health education specialist should emphasize cost savings rather than costs.

53. D: If the health education specialist hires a consultant to install hardware and software as part of program implementation, the health education specialist should prepare a statement of work (SOW). The SOW is frequently used in project management to ensure that the consultant understands the specific tasks and the expected timeline for completion of the work. The SOW should outline the purpose of the project, the type of work to be done, the location, the time period, deliverables, standards that must be met, payment schedule, criteria for acceptance, and any special requirements.

54. D: Based on the national statistics in the graph, the ethnic group of boys 12 to 19 that showed the greatest increase in obesity between 1994 and 2009 is Mexican Americans. While the percentage of increase in non-Hispanic whites rose for 11.6% to 17.5% for a total increase of 5.9%, the percentage increase for non-Hispanic blacks rose from 10.7 % to 22.6% for an overall increase of 11.9%. Mexican Americans showed the highest beginning rate and the highest ending rate, rising from 14.8% to 28.9% with an overall increase of 14.8%.

55. B: Considering the information in the graph that shows that Mexican American adolescent males have the highest rates of obesity according to national statistics, the next step to take if developing a program to fight adolescent obesity is to obtain local statistics about adolescent obesity. While national statistics can be used for benchmarking, the health education specialist cannot assume that the national statistics mirror the local population because that may or may not be true, depending on many different factors.

56. C: "What interventions should be instituted?" is not an appropriate question to ask during the first step of a needs assessment because it is too early in the process to begin considering interventions, and doing so may bias the findings. The health education specialist should be considering the scope of assessment and such issues as goals of the needs assessment, the resources needed to carry out the assessment, and how extensive the needs assessment should be.

57. A: When extracting data from a database using Boolean operators, if the health education specialist wants to retrieve documents that contain information about hypertension associated with obesity among adolescent African Americans, the most appropriate search is: hypertension AND adolescent AND obesity AND African American. This search will produce documents that contain all four of these key terms. The operator OR would produce documents that contain one term or the other but not necessarily both. The operator NOT may eliminate too many documents, such as those with comparison data.

58. D: The first issue to consider when determining the validity of data is the source. If the source is not valid, then the data should not be used. Valid sources include juried journals and government websites, such as the CDC. If the data are from the Internet, URLs ending in .gov are likely to provide valid data. URLs ending in .org may be valid, but the organization should be researched. Valid information may also be found with URLs ending in .edu, but in some cases all staff and students can use .edu, so not all information may be valid.

59. B: If the health education specialist conducted a survey to determine how many employees smoke in the workplace but wants more information about smoking behavior, the best method of data collection is probably observation. The health education specialist may observe the number and frequency of visits to a smoking area on an individual basis as well as totals for the employees. Studies have shown that people often under report smoking behavior, assuming that they spend less time smoking than they actually do.

60. D: Reasons to train personnel who are assisting with data collection include to prevent ethics violations by reviewing ethical considerations, to ensure timely data collection by providing instruction and practice in procedures, and (most importantly) to ensure consistency because data are not valid if collected in different manners. One can never guarantee accurate analysis although that should certainly be the aim, but analysis is a concern for after data are collected, not before.

61. A: The primary problem with using only community forums to gather data about a priority population is that the forum members may not be representative of the population as a whole. People who participate in community forums are often better informed and more active in the community in general, but they may not represent the views of the silent majority who do not participate. For this reason, alternate methods of gathering data should be considered to supplement data derived from community forums.

62. B: If a state with a large undocumented immigrant population has prohibited the use of public funds to provide healthcare for this population, the impact of this legislation is likely increased disease and disability. Undocumented immigrants are often fearful of the authorities and often go without medical care, and free clinics are not always available or not easily accessible to a population that may lack adequate transportation or may work long hours.

63. B: If the health education specialist is interested in conducting legislative lobbying about a number of health-related issues, the health education specialist should begin by focusing on one issue. The health education specialist should study the issue in depth and go to the legislators with a fact list as well as a list of questions. The health education should also study the record of the legislators and know their positions on issues and voting records.

64. C: According to the Joint Committee on Standards for Educational Evaluation, the standard that means that information gathered in evaluation must serve the needs of those who will use the information is *utility*. Feasibility, on the other hand, means that the process used must be realistic and prudent as well as frugal and diplomatic. Propriety refers to legal and ethical behavior on the part of evaluator, and accuracy means that the finding must provide information that is accurate.

65. B: The purpose of an outcome chain is to help identify long and short-term outcomes leading to attainment of goals. The outcome chain identifies the different types of responses expected from the project/program. Example: Information and demonstration will lead to RESPONSE (customer feedback regarding usefulness) → KNOWLEDGE (learning achieved) → BEHAVIOR (changes associated with learning) → OUTCOMES (improvements) → GOAL ACHIEVEMENT (benefits and evident results).

66. B: If the health education specialist is implementing an education program about sexually transmitted diseases (STDs) and has set a goal that within one year there will be no further cases of STDs among adolescents, the potential problem that may arise is that the goal is unrealistic. By setting the goal at zero (0), the health education specialist is setting the stage for failure by establishing expectations that cannot generally be met.

67. A: If the health education specialist needs more information about the sexual activity of adolescents in the school district in order to better plan program strategies, the best method to obtain this information is probably in-class anonymous surveys because mailed surveys tend to have a low response rate, focus groups review strategies already in place, and student-led discussion groups don't provide adequate confidentiality and may not provide a representative group or reliable information.

68. A: If the health education specialist is planning a delivery method to educate adolescents about the dangers of unprotected sexual activity and different types of sexually transmitted diseases, the best method of delivery is probably a computer video game. Computer video games are extremely popular with this age group, which has essentially grown up with computers and video games. Computer video games engage the adolescents and require interaction and decision-making, and these actions can help to facilitate learning.

69. C: Public forums are often used to obtain qualitative statistics. Other qualitative methods include the use of key informants to learn information about a priority population, informal interviews (person on the street), and focus groups. Qualitative methods are used to elicit feelings, beliefs, and opinions, and this subjective information may provide valuable insight into problems, gaps in services, or barriers to implementation of a program. In most cases, both qualitative and quantitative methods are used for assessment.

70. B: If using the FOG index to assess readability so that material can be adapted for consumers, the health education specialist should first count the number of words and the number of sentences in a passage, ensuring that the passage is 100 words in length. The average sentence length (ASL) is obtained by dividing the number of sentences into the number of words. Next, the 3-syllable or more words are counted (excluding proper nouns, hyphenated words, and words made 3 syllables by the addition of –es or –ed suffixes). This number is divided by the total number of words and converted to a percentage to find the percentage of hard words (PHW). The ASL and PHW are added together and multiplied by 0.4 to find the approximate grade level of the material.

71. D: The best use of a focus group is to provide a response to proposed interventions prior to implementation. The focus group may identify problems with the interventions or possible barriers to implementation. Focus groups are usually comprised of 10 to 15 people, who should be representative of the priority population. The leader of the focus group, sometimes a paid professional, is responsible for guiding the discussion and obtaining useful information. Sessions are usually limited to about an hour with only 5 or 6 questions or issues addressed in a session.

72. A: According to *Healthy People 2020*, one aspect of the key area *social and communication context* of social determinants is incarceration/ institutionalization. Other aspects include social cohesion, participation in civic events, and perceptions of discrimination and/or equity. Other key areas include economic stability (stability of housing, poverty levels, employment, food security), education (graduation rates, literacy, enrollment in higher education), health and health care (access to health care, health literacy), and neighborhood and built environment (access to healthy food, quality housing, environmental conditions, crime and violence).

73. B: Health illiteracy is an example of a societal factor. The Prevention Institute has identified four categories of factors that are root cases of racial and ethnic disparities: societal (poverty health illiteracy, educational deficits, economics, racism), environmental (unsafe social/environmental environments, exposure to toxins and pathogenic organisms, inadequate access to food, limited exercise options, community norms), individual/behavioral (lifestyle choices), and medical care (limited access, poor quality, inadequate cultural competence of caregivers).

74. C: Social networks and norms are part of the community level of influence of health behaviors. The individual level includes personal attitudes, beliefs, and knowledge while the interpersonal level includes associations with family, friends, and peers that help to define social identity and roles. The institutional level includes the rules, regulations, and policies that may serve as a barrier or support for recommended behavior. The public policy level relates to local, state, and national policies and laws that support interventions.

75. C: If, when planning interventions for a priority population in which the eldest male in the family makes the decisions, the health education specialist determines that this method of decision making is counter to American ideals and plans to focus on empowering the women in the population to make independent decisions, this is an example of ethnocentrism. With ethnocentrism, an individual believes that his or her practices or beliefs are the only correct ones and that others should follow this model.

76. D: If, when designing interventions for a health promotion, the health education specialist plans a multi-level approach in order to allow any member of the priority population who wants to participate the opportunity to do so, the ethical principle that the health education is applying to this strategy is *equity*. Equity involves not only equal access to a program but can also include *demand equity* in which access is according to need as well as *supply equity*, in which each individual is allotted an equal measure of resources.

77. C: If using the PRECEDE-PROCEED planning model to guide the delivery of a health promotion plan, administrative and policy assessment is completed in phase 4, the first phase of the PROCEED portion. Phase 5 is implementation of the program, Phase 6 is process evaluation, phase 7 is impact evaluation, and phase 5 is outcome evaluation. The PRECEDE-PROCEED model focuses on assessment and evaluation. The PRECEDE portion has 3 phases. Phase 1 is social assessment of the priority population, phase 2 is epidemiological assessment of the population, and phase 3 is educational and ecological assessment.

78. A: An example of an intangible resource for an organization is the organization's image. Other intangible resources may include patents and intellectual property. Human resources are usually the most valuable and can include staff members, community members, partners, and volunteers. Tangible resources are usually considered those things with a physical presence, such as equipment, paper, and books. The health education specialist should carefully consider the resources available and the resources needed during the process of program planning.

79. B: The time estimates utilized in a Program Evaluation and Review Technique (PERT) chart do not include anticipated time. The PERT chart utilizes four different time estimates:

Optimistic time: The shortest period of time in which the activity can be carried out.

Most likely time: The time period that has the highest degree of probability.

Pessimistic time: The longest time period that may be required to complete an activity.

Expected time: Calculated using the formula: (optimistic time plus 4 X the most likely time plus the pessimistic time) divided by 6.

80. C: If soliciting feedback about an education program, the method that will likely provide the best response rate is providing printed surveys directly to participants during the program and providing time for them to fill them out and turn them in. Valuable information may also be gained by asking participants, but some people are not comfortable expressing their opinions verbally, especially if the opinions are negative. Email and mail surveys tend to have low response rates.

81. A: The primary purpose of carrying out a feasibility study is to identify factors that may interfere with implementation. The format of the study may vary according to the type of program but should consider such factors as funding and whether or not it is adequate to sustain the program, resources available and needed (including human resources), and policies or regulations that may preclude the program (such as a needle distribution program where laws prohibit such a program).

82. D: "Education is free from discrimination and harassment" is not a part of Article V, Responsibility in Research and Evaluation, of the Code of Ethics for the Health Education Profession as it applies to Article I, Responsibility in Professional Preparation. Article 5 focuses on ensuring that the Health Education Specialist conducts research or evaluation in compliance with applicable laws, regulation, policies, and professional standards. Article 5 includes doing no harm, ensuring voluntary participation, and sharing conflicts of interest.

83. B: When communicating findings to partners and stakeholders through a written report, the data analysis plan should be described in the methodology section. While papers vary somewhat, they usually begin with an introduction that provides an overview followed by a literature review that describes relevant studies and theories. The next section is methodology, which should describe in detail how research was conducted. The results section provides the findings, and the conclusion indicates whether the hypothesis was supported or not.

84. C: A health impact assessment (HIA) should generally be carried out before development or implementation. The purpose of the HIA is to determine the potential health effects of a possible program. Initially, screening should be done to determine if the HIA is indicated and then scoping to determine the health effects to consider. Both the risks and benefits of the program or policy should be considered when developing recommendations to promote positive effects or mitigate negative ones.

85. D: If findings of a pilot study to increase screening for domestic abuse show markedly inconsistent results depending on when and by whom the screening is carried out, the first factor to consider is training. Consistency is critical to any program, and when the results vary depending on the person doing the screening, then the most common reason is that the training has been inadequate or the people who are trained are not using the proper protocol.

86. A: AHRQ Innovations Exchange provides access to a wide range of evidence-based approaches that may apply to public health with links to evidence-based guides from other sites, such as SAMSHA. The purpose of the site is to facilitate change and adapting of new evidence-based approaches to the delivery of healthcare. The website provides searchable innovations and tools, articles and resources and opportunities to network with innovators and organizations.

87. C: When sending an email to communicate with a priority population, the health education specialist should be aware that the primary determinant in whether the person reads the email or not is often the subject line. Because people often scan through emails quickly when deciding what to read, the subject line should be short (no more than 50 characters) and to the point. Words in upper case (electronic shouting) and special characters should be avoided when possible.

88. A: If the health education specialist has located a data collection instrument that seems appropriate but has a readability level that is far too high for the priority population, which has low literacy rates, the health education specialist should attempt to locate a different instrument. Altering the items on an instrument to change the readability level may substantially change the validity and reliability of the instrument. As a last resort, the health education specialist may need to construct an instrument, but this is often a time-consuming and difficult process in order to ensure reliability and validity.

89. B: If the health education specialist would like to utilize smart phones to communicate with and send information to members of a priority population, the first step should be to survey the population regarding smart phone use. If some members of the priority population do not have smart phones, this may pose the ethical problem of equity if a suitable alternative cannot be determined. Once the survey is completed and the health education specialist has data, a decision can be made about the appropriateness of using smart phones.

90. D: If the health education specialist works for a large industrial corporation and is selecting technology to manage program data for a health initiative, the first step should be to assess existing technology and resources. If the technology purchased is different from that used by the corporation, then this may entail the need for additional funds for training, software, and staff. The health education specialist should also determine if existing technology can be used or if new equipment could be utilized for additional purposes.

91. D: The most important factor in ensuring consistency in implementation of a health education program is usually training. Staff and volunteers should be thoroughly trained in processes and in the use of the materials and have practice time under observation. If the program is designed so that handbooks or guides are utilized instead of direct training, then they should be clearly written and detailed and, when possible, video demonstrations should be provided.

92. B: If the health education specialist plans to monitor computer use, the first step is to provide a written policy. Staff members should be very clear about what they can and cannot do on the computers and should be made aware that use will be monitored, how monitoring will be done, and how information will be secured. If email or access to social media is allowed, then acceptable use should also be spelled out (usually prohibiting threatening, obscene, or sexually-explicit messages).

93. C: When conducting a survey as part of a needs assessment the type of survey that is likely to have the lowest response rate is a telephone survey. Telephone surveys usually have about an 8 to 12% return, about half of that achieved by most mail or email surveys although this may vary somewhat according to population. One major problem with telephoned surveys is that many people have caller ID and don't pick up the phone for surveys or let calls go to voicemail.

94. C: If the health education specialist wants to establish a resource database that includes resources that may aid in the development of the program regarding misuse of alcohol and medications among older adults, the first step should be to determine the type of resources needed, being as concrete as possible. Data collection of any type should not be done randomly but rather with purpose so that the search can be focused and more productive. Resources may include individuals, organizations, agencies, businesses, and/or facilities.

95. A: If the health education specialist plans to present workshops at senior citizen's centers and retirement homes about the signs of alcohol and medication misuse and the presentation includes a

141

20-minute video, which will be preceded by an introduction of the main points of the video, the most valuable use of time following the video is to have a discussion period, usually ranging from 10 to 40 minutes. This allows participants to more easily recall material in the video about which they have questions or comments.

96. B: If an older adult asks about an article about medication misuse in a popular magazine, wondering if the information that summarizes a study done by a university is valid, the health education specialist should offer to research the primary source of information about the study. While valid information is often reported in the popular press, it is sometimes written about inaccurately or written so that information can be misconstrued. This presents a good opportunity to discuss the importance of getting information from valid sources.

97. D: If the health education specialist has been unable to find appropriate materials for a priority population of non-Spanish-speaking indigenous Mayan immigrants from Guatemala and has, therefore, developed handouts, checklists, and guides independently with the help of a professional translator, before full implementation, the health education specialist should pilot test the materials on a small group. Whenever possible, the health education specialist should use materials that have already been validated. Pilot testing allows the health education specialist to modify the materials as needed.

98. A: If the health education specialist has convinced the school to place only healthy snacks in the vending machines when implementing a program to improve student nutrition and reduce obesity, but the result has been a sharp decline in purchases from the vending machines because the students are unhappy with the choices, this is an example of *reciprocal determinism.* This means that although environmental factors (such as the change in foods in the vending machines) influence individuals and their behavior, the individuals can also regulate their own behavior (by not purchasing the foods).

99. D: An example of a tailored message is an Internet pop-up as with health information based on the individual's Internet searches. Tailored messages are individualized in such a way that they appear to be personal although they may be computer-generated according to algorithms. Information or assumptions about the person are used to generate the message content. One of the primary purposes of a tailored message is to make the recipient more receptive to the message.

100. B: If the health education specialist has placed information about self-breast exam on a website and wants to determine if information has been viewed by an adequate number of people, the best method is to use a web counter to track traffic to the website. Some web counters can track, for example, the duration of time that a viewer paused on a page and how long the session was. Often only a small percentage of people are willing to complete a survey, and obtaining information about mammograms or from local practitioners may be hard to obtain and may be unrelated to viewing.

101. C: If, as part of a program to decrease violence in the schools, the health education specialist has been educating staff and students about the use of messaging and other social media to intimidate, threaten, and damage the reputation of students and faculty, this type of behavior is classified as electronic aggression, which can involve any type of technology. Electronic aggression has driven some students to suicide or severe depression, so it is a major concern in schools.

102. D: If the health education specialist is a member of the curriculum committee in a school district and helps to select health topics and instructional materials but has received dozens of books, pamphlets, and other materials from publishers and government agencies to review, the first step should be to develop or find a materials review form so that there is consistency to the review. The review form should contain such categories as the type of material, readability, and cost. If computerized, then sorting according to specific criteria (such as readability or cost) can be done rapidly.

103. D: When enrolling patients in a heart healthy program to help them better control their blood pressure and cholesterol levels through diet, exercise, and lifestyle changes, the first action should be to gather baseline data, such as blood pressure, pulse, and weight and other demographic information. Baseline data is especially important as a point of reference to determine if the patients are making progress. It's important to maintain privacy during data collection, as people are often especially sensitive about weight.

104. A: If the health education specialist finds as the date of implementation of a new program nears that one important component of the project has lagged behind and will not be fully completed by the target date, the best solution is to delay implementation. A program is often as strong as its weakest component, so starting a new program before it is fully ready is not likely to result in the expected outcomes and may negatively affect the program as a whole.

105. B: While there are many advantages to the lecture format for teaching (cost saving, time saving) a group of participants in a health education program, one limitation is that the health education specialist is delivering exactly the same information to all of the group members without being able to individualize the lesson. This is especially a problem with a heterogeneous group whose members may have different levels of health literacy. If using a lecture format, the health education specialist should plan time for questions and answers or discussion periods.

106. D: Regardless of the demographics of a priority population, when assessing readiness for implementation of an organization's health promotion plan, the health education specialist should focus on available resources and leadership commitment. Without adequate resources, both tangible (equipment, staff, volunteers) and intangible (motivation, support, organization culture), a program cannot function; and without leadership commitment, a program cannot be sustained. Support from leadership helps to engender support from others within an organization.

107. A: When utilizing direct mailing part of a marketing plan, the best method is likely targeted mailing in which mailings are made to those who meet specific criteria. Mass mailing can become quite expensive because of postage costs, and the mailings will, in many cases, be wasted on people with no interest. Mailing to key informants alone is usually not adequate although doing so may aid the marketing campaign. Mailing marketing materials on request reaches a very limited population.

108. C: When implementing a worksite health promotion effort that includes hiring and managing personnel, the best way to avoid conflict in the workplace is by clearly outlining expectations in terms of time, appearance, demeanor, inclusiveness, confidentiality, and interactions with others. Personnel should be aware of any rules or regulations that apply to their positions and should understand disciplinary procedures. It's better to take the time to avoid conflict than to manage it.

109. D: If, when applying the Theory of Planned Behavior in a program to decrease smoking among adolescents, the health education specialist recruits coaches, teachers, and student leaders that the adolescents respect to encourage smoking cessation, this is an example of utilizing the construct of *subjective norm*. Adolescents, especially, may be influenced by those whom they value, and this is important to remember when planning programs and interventions for adolescents. Attitude toward behavior refers to the adolescent's personal attitude, such as a positive or negative attitude toward quitting.

110. A: If the health education specialist wants to use social modeling according to the concepts of Social Cognitive Theory (SCT) to influence students at a university to develop strategies to avoid situations in which date rape may occur, the health education specialist needs to find student peers to talk about strategies and methods they use to avoid date rape. SCT focuses on psychological and environmental determinants of behavior and the power of observational learning and self-regulation. If students see that their peers act to prevent date rape, this increases their self-efficacy and ability to regulate their own behavior.

111. C: The Rapid Estimate of Adult Literacy in Medicine (REALM) instrument to assess health literacy requires that people read through 3 lists of common medical terms and lay terms for body parts and disorders. The people are advised to read as many words as possible in the lists with no more than 5 seconds allotted for each word. Correct words are given one point with no points for words that are missed or mispronounced. Total score is used to estimate approximate grade level:

0 to 18: up to 3rd grade.

19 to 44: 4th to 6th grade.

45 to 60: 7th to 8th grade.

61 to 66: 9th to 12th grade.

Greater than 66: Above high school.

112. C: If utilizing the Health Belief Model (HBM) as the basis for a communication strategy to increase participation in smoking cessation programs, the health education specialist must survey to find perceptions about smoking. Then, communication is targeted toward those perceptions. The HBM is based on a number of constructs:

Perceived susceptibility: belief about the likelihood of getting a disease.

Perceived severity: seriousness of contracting a disease.

Perceived benefits: benefits of change in behavior to decrease the likelihood of disease.

Perceived barriers: negative aspects of a change in behavior.

113. B: Key informants of a priority population are usually those in positions of power or influence. These may include community leaders, legislators, and spiritual leaders (ministers, priests, rabbis, imams). Gaining the cooperation and support of key informants is often critical to acceptance, especially in communities with ethnic populations with limited English language skills or mistrust of authorities. Key informant interviews may provide much valuable and detailed information about a priority population.

114. A: While learning skills, such as monitoring diabetes and injecting insulin utilizes the cognitive (knowledge, recall) and psychomotor (physical skills) domains of learning, the affective (feeling) domain should be assessed first because an individual's ability to learn and motivation to carry out tasks are often most influenced by feelings and attitudes. If a person feels very negatively about having diabetes and is stressed and upset, the ability to learn is significantly impaired.

115. C: A health education specialist who understands the importance of building relationships with many individuals in a priority population and encouraging people to work together is interested in investing in social capital. Developing networks between community members helps to build trust and to engage them in the process of change. When people know each other and have established relationships for links in society, and these networks of people are more likely to cooperate and achieve results.

116. B: A focus group is a small group of individuals who are selected based on certain similarities such as age, stage in life, or place of residence. Trying to set up a focus group with certain similarities helps to keep individuals from feeling intimidated by others' opinions. Multiple focus groups can be set up using different types. The focus group is led by a moderator or facilitator who poses certain questions to the group involving strengths, issues, concerns, or other topics to be discussed. The facilitator should lead the discussion and try to help the group stay on topic but try to remain in the background so people can talk freely. Opinions are collected, and the information that is obtained is subjective and not statistically valid. Once the focus group is finished, the information can be compiled based on the questions that were discussed then categorized within each question. The information that is obtained can be the start of the needs assessment.

117. A: When conducting a needs assessment, sources of health-related data can be obtained from two areas. Primary data are collected using techniques such as interview, observation of the population being studied, community forums, questionnaires, or a self-assessment tool. Secondary data sources include obtaining data from government agencies such as the Centers for Disease Control and Prevention, United States Census Bureau, or the Department of Health and Human Services. Secondary data can also be obtained from state or local agencies that keep various types of vital records or statistics such as morbidity or mortality records, disease registries, or police records. Nongovernment agencies such as hospitals can provide various types of secondary data such as information on discharges. Peer-reviewed journals or scientific studies are also sources of secondary data.

118. D: There are many factors that may help to improve or hinder the health of a community. Biological factors such as genetics are important to address but may be less effective as part of a large group. Lifestyle factors such as increased rates of smoking, poor diet, or alcohol use have a direct impact on the health of a community. Environmental factors can include issues such as access to affordable food or health care, air quality, or water quality. Psychosocial factors may include availability of social supports, employment, income level, education level, or overall safety of the community. Other types of individual factors may include religious or cultural beliefs.

119. A: There are typically six steps in the needs assessment process. The first step is to determine why the needs assessment is being done and the scope of the project. The second step is gathering the data, followed by data analysis. The fourth step is to look at any factors that have been identified as having an impact on the health issue. The fifth step is to determine what the actual focus should be for addressing the health problem. The last step is to validate the needs that have been identified. This makes sure that the identified issue is a true need.

120. C: A face-to-face survey would be the most expensive type of survey to use because it is time consuming. Less expensive options include mail, telephone, or Internet surveys. Face-to-face surveys have a higher response rate than other types of surveys, but they increase interviewer bias and take away the option of a participant to remain anonymous. With a face-to-face interview, the surveyor is able to ask questions in the desired order, and it allows for additional questioning or asking for clarification if necessary. It is more difficult to summarize the data for face-to-face surveys.

121. B: A clinical indicator is a type of secondary data that can be utilized as part of existing health records. A clinical indicator measures the outcome of care. It should be designed in a way that alerts a clinician to a certain event. A clinical indicator does not provide an answer to an issue but instead flags a problem that needs to be addressed. It provides a way to identify issues that need to be improved upon. Clinical indicators can be compared against national benchmarks. An example of a clinical indicator that a health education specialist may use would be body mass index values for an elementary school to determine obesity rates.

122. A: When planning a health education program, it is important to obtain support from members of the community in order to increase the chances that the program will be a success. The support should come from key leaders or members of the community including local politicians, members of the clergy, or local health agencies. It is also important to involve members associated with the population that is being targeted such as individuals who are directly affected or leaders within that population. Community groups should also be approached to obtain commitment to the health education program. A planning committee can be established utilizing individuals from the various groups, and a group leader should be selected.

123. B: The needs assessment identified the increased rate of low-birth-weight (LBW) infants as an area that needs to be addressed through health education. It is important to know the risk factors for delivering an LBW infant in order to develop the most effective goal for the program. Some of the risk factors for low-birth-weight infants include lack of prenatal care, history of previous LBW infant, chronic maternal health issues, smoking during pregnancy, poor weight gain, minority women with low income levels, teen pregnancies, and spacing of children too close together. Of the goals listed above, targeting Caucasian women of normal childbearing age would have the least effect on reducing the incidence of low-birth-weight infants.

124. D: It is difficult to teach people who do not want to learn. There are a number of strategies that can be employed to maximize the learning process. Individuals are least likely to retain information if they only read it, hear it, or see it. They are much more likely to retain information when they hear and see what is being presented (50%). Using audiovisual aids such as PowerPoint is important to contribute to the learning process. Individuals also need to be actively involved such as participating in discussions instead of just listening to a lecture. Repetition is important as well remembering to summarize important points from time to time. Helping the participants to understand why the information is important to them is also a key factor in the learning process. Information should not be provided too quickly but should be adjusted to the level of the audience.

125. B: The PRECEDE-PROCEED model was initially developed in the 1970s and was revised in the 1980s to include five additional phases. There are nine phases altogether in this planning model for health education that apply to the priority population. Phase 1 is social assessment where the quality of life of the population being addressed is examined. Phase 2 is epidemiological assessment where the heath issues are examined. Behavioral and environmental assessment is the third phase risk factors associated where the health problems are identified. Phase 4 is the educational and ecological assessment where various behaviors are identified. Phase 5 is the administrative and policy assessment where resources are identified for the program. Phase 6 is implementation. Phases 7, 8, and 9 are the process, impact, and outcome evaluations.

126. C: MATCH is an acronym for Mobilizing Action Toward Community Health. The MATCH model is a community-based, multilevel model that utilizes five phases. Within each phase, there are several steps. The first phase is selection of goals, taking into account prevalence, population, and behavioral and environmental goals. The second phase is intervention planning, which takes into account the targets of the intervention, objectives, mediators, and the approaches to be used. The third phase of MATCH is program development, which creates the components of the program; develops the curriculum, learning objectives, and materials to be used; and develops the session plans and materials. The fourth phase is implementation preparations where individuals are trained as implementers and ways to help make implementation easier are identified. The last phase is evaluation where the process is evaluated, the impact of the program is determined, and outcomes are monitored.

127. D: There are many different types of objectives associated with a health program. Learning objectives are also known as instructional objectives, and these are short-term, measurable points that are directly related to the material that is being taught. For a program that is trying to provide education on saturated fat in the diet, the ability to correctly identify three sources of saturated fat in the diet would be an example of a learning objective. Other types of objectives include outcome objectives, which directly related to the goals of the program and are measurable. Outcome objectives are considered the endpoint of a program. Behavioral objectives describe the behaviors that the program is trying to address. Reduction of the specific behavior will lead to the achievement of the program goal. Objectives need to be written as clearly defined statements that include only one indicator or issue. A reasonable time frame should be identified. A way to measure the criteria must also be identified.

128. A: An environmental objective is a nonbehavioral objective that addresses changes in the environment to improve the health or behavior of the population. Environmental factors can include physical factors such as air quality, pollution, waste management, hazardous waste disposal, water quality, or noise. It can also include social factors such as cultural, religious, economic, or political resources. Psychological factors are also included such as support systems. Environmental objectives can be looked at as a way of removing the physical or social obstacles that prevent changes in behavior from occurring. The evaluation of the environmental objective would be to determine if the change in environment helped improve health.

129. D: In order for a health education plan to be effective, all factors that may hinder or promote compliance must be examined prior to implementation. If there is a high percentage of residents in this rural community that utilize food stamps, one may infer that money for extras such as health club membership is not plentiful. In order to encourage residents to join a health club, the cost must not be prohibitive. Obtaining insurance coverage, corporate sponsorships, or other ways to reduce fees would be worth looking into. Community or school competitions may be fun, low-cost ways to encourage involvement to the program. Certainly utilizing the outdoors is also a great way to encourage exercise. Providing seminars or in-services at no cost to participants would be a great way to teach people about healthful eating on a budget. It is important to identify and address any obstacles in order to make a health education program successful.

130. C: A community garden would likely be most effective in a local setting such as a town or city. It would be a way to encourage consumption of fresh vegetables in a low-cost and interesting way. A health educator in a college or university setting may teach a health class or find ways to promote healthful eating in the cafeteria. In a business setting, a health educator may try to address health needs of employees, which may be obtained through surveys. Topics may include smoking cessation, healthful eating, or stress reduction. In the healthcare setting, classes targeting specific issues may be offered such as weight reduction or lowering cholesterol levels. It is important for the health educator to be aware of the specific setting and utilize appropriate materials based on the target audience.

131. B: A pretest is a useful tool for assessing the group that is being targeted for health education. Knowledge and attitudes can be assessed as well as the skill level of the group. A pretest helps to determine the comprehension level of the group as a whole and can help determine how to gear the information. Overall strengths and weaknesses can be determined, which can also help to gear the material appropriately. A pretest can also help to identify any cultural or religious issues that may be pertinent. A pretest cannot be the tool that ensures changes in behavior or initiates the education process.

132. B: Cultural competence is where diversity is valued and is demonstrated by providing a safe and welcoming environment for people from various cultural and ethnic backgrounds. Cultural competence is not something that can be taught but rather is developed over a period of time. This may include program policies, standards of care, behaviors, or attitudes. An example of cultural competence would be hiring bilingual employees who are involved in the education process. There are three steps involved in becoming culturally competent. The first is developing awareness of one's own values or beliefs about various cultures. The second is acquiring knowledge in order to understand other cultures and how other cultures view themselves. The third step is to develop and maintain cross-cultural skills that can be applied to the population being addressed. Cultural sensitivity is a part of cultural competence but is more about knowing that both differences and similarities exist between groups but values are not assigned to either.

133. A: Instructional technology is a very important part of a health educator's job. Knowledge of basic computer software, such as word processing, spreadsheets, and PowerPoint, is essential to effective job performance. Email remains an important communication tool along with other technology such as texting and blogs. Social networking sites are also becoming important tools for education, including Facebook and Twitter. It is essential that the health educator have a working knowledge of this type of media. The ability to use introductory statistical software packages is also important in the health educator's job. The use of search engines is essential to job performance; however, it is the responsibility of the health educator to be able to effectively utilize these search engines and be able to determine whether a Web site has reputable information or not.

134. B: There are typically five phases that occur during the implementation of a health education program. The first phase is gaining acceptance of a program. This needs to be accomplished with the priority population that will be the target of the program as well as the sponsors of the program and the employees who will staff the program. All of these individuals or groups must be on board in the initial phase in order to be successful. Much of this phase can be accomplished in the needs assessment portion if the assessment was done properly. The second phase is to develop an estimation of the resources required such as space, supplies, money, or equipment and to identify tasks that need to be accomplished. The third is to develop a system for managing the program including a schedule, staff involved, and finances. The fourth phase is implementing the program. The last phase is to decide if or when the program will end or if the program will continue indefinitely.

135. D: There are three ways a health education program can be set into action. The first is pilot testing or field testing. This is when a program is tested out in a small group with individuals who are similar to the priority population being targeted with the program. For example, if you are testing a diabetes prevention program, the program may be piloted with individuals who are overweight and with a borderline blood glucose level. The second way is phasing in. This is when the total program is broken up into parts then each part is introduced at a separate time. The program can be divided by the number of participants able to enroll at one time or offering a program at one location at a time. The third way to put a program into action is total implementation, in which an entire program is introduced simultaneously. This may be done for a program that deals with one topic only though a single lecture or a weight loss challenge.

136. A: There are many theories or models used in education that help to address the potential issues in program delivery. The transtheoretical model is also known as the stages of change model.

This model helps to identify a particular stage that an individual is in with regard to the changes they need to make in a certain behavior. The stages include precontemplation, contemplation, preparation, action, maintenance, and termination. A person can be in one specific stage but can move back and forth between stages very easily. It is important to identify the correct stage in order to maximize the learning potential or to be able to recognize if the person just isn't ready to learn, making any attempts at education futile at the moment. It may also direct how the education may be addressed.

137. C: This man is currently in the preparation phase, in which there is intent to make changes within the next month. This is evidenced by his selection of a quit date within three weeks and an upcoming appointment to look into nicotine replacement therapy. If he was in the precontemplation phase, he would have no desire to quit smoking at this moment. If he was in the contemplation phase, he would be looking at making a plan within a six-month timeframe. If he was in the action phase, he would have already refrained from smoking consistently but for less than six months. If he was in the maintenance phase, he would be smoke free for more than six months. In the termination phase, he would have no temptation at all to resume smoking.

138. D: Informed consent is the procedure used to explain various facets of a program or treatment. As it pertains to a health program, informed consent may include the possible risks and potential benefits, the purpose of the program, and any possible side effects or inconveniences of participation. Informed consent also provides an individual with the ability to stop the program at any time. Informed consent may also include other ways for an individual to obtain similar health benefits. An informed consent should be a written document that is signed by the participant.

139. B: Preventable chronic diseases can cost employers and taxpayers quite a bit of money. By implementing companywide wellness programs, employers can not only significantly reduce the health risks of their employees and improve the quality of life, but they can also reduce healthcare costs significantly and improve productivity by reducing absenteeism. This in turn can financially be passed on to the employees by lowering health insurance premiums. It is difficult for people to make changes, and just offering wellness programs or informational newsletters does not induce change. Mandating participation is also not a good idea. The best way to promote participation would be to make participation as easy as possible. This would include mobile or on-site screenings with added monetary incentives such as receiving gift cards for participating and continuing with follow-ups.

140. C: It is important to know the target group that the health education program is planned for. Different strategies work better for some groups than for others. In a middle-school age group of adolescents, it is important to refrain from trying to increase student knowledge by talking about scientific facts and theories. This age group needs to have tangible information that they can relate directly to themselves and to their peers. The information being presented needs to be goal oriented with specific behavioral objectives identified. The information does need to be research based; however, it is best presented when related to social factors, attitudes, behaviors, or skills of the group. The adolescents will need to be able to weigh the information being received against how it will affect their own life or those around them. They need to be able to assess risks and benefits as well as how to get out of certain situations they may be confronted with.

141. B: When preparing to present a lecture, remember that the average length of an individual's attention span is about 12 to 20 minutes without interruptions. If a longer lecture is planned, it is better to divide it into smaller 15- to 20-minute segments in order to maximize focus. This can be done by introducing questions after each segment or incorporating a group activity. Utilizing notes is also more effective than reading from a preplanned script. Visual aids can help to keep individuals focused on the lecture, and sometimes it is more helpful to give handouts at the end of the session rather than before, but the audience should be aware of this so they do not spend a lot of extra time and effort trying to write everything down. In the case of PowerPoint slides, it may be more useful to provide copies of the slides to allow participants to take notes as you move through the slides.

142. D: URL stands for "uniform resource locator." Quite a bit of useful information can be obtained just by looking at the URL of a Web site. It does not give an indication if any of the information is safe, valid, or correct. It can identify if the Web site belongs to a certain individual because the person's name will be listed with a tilde (~) or a percent sign beside their name. It may also indicate using "users" or "members." The URL will also indicate if the server is using a commercial ISP or is using a Web page hosting service, such as AOL. The domain will also be listed. A domain of ".gov" indicates a government Web site, ".edu" indicates an educational Web site, and ".org" indicates a nonprofit organization. A domain of ".com" indicates a commercial Web site and will need closer scrutiny pertaining to the accuracy of the information. The publisher of the Web site is usually listed as part of the Web address and is located just after "http://."

143. C: A randomized controlled trial is considered the gold standard for research design. This type of trial randomly assigns subjects to either the control group or the intervention group. The end results of the intervention are then measured. The randomization factor helps the researcher to evaluate whether the effects are due to the actual intervention instead of other factors such as age or socioeconomic status. When evaluating research, it is important to look at the quality of the evidence in terms of being a randomized controlled trial as well as a trial that is well designed. The planned intervention should be clearly identified as well as who is providing the intervention and how the control group and the intervention group are different. Any sort of crossover from one group into the other should be identified and evaluated as well. Any outcome measures that are used need to be validated. Data about long-term results are also important to determine if the intervention was effective over a period of time.

144. D: The IRB is an institutional review board. Federal law requires that any institution conducting research that involves living people must establish an IRB that provides initial approval to the study as well as to monitor the research throughout its trial to ensure that human rights are protected. The IRB typically consists of physicians, researchers, members of the community, and statisticians. The IRB makes sure that the type of research being done is ethical and that no harm will come to the study participants. The Food and Drug Administration is responsible for the monitoring of all the individual IRBs to ensure compliance with federal law.

145. A: Descriptive statistics involves the use of tables, graphs, charts, and numbers to organize data. It is used to look at the location of data and where the data fall. It looks at the variability of data (dispersion) and measures the variance and standard deviation. It also looks at the symmetrical pattern of the data (skew) as well as the peakedness (kurtosis) of the data. Variables are quantities or qualities and are divided into three groups: nominal (names or categories), ordinal (order or rank of the variables), and interval variables (numeric).

146. B: The measure of central tendency is the location of data as measured by the mean, median, and mode. The mean refers to the average of the data and is most commonly used. It does not, however, always provide the best depiction of the results because data on either the upper or lower extreme will raise or lower the average in a manner inconsistent with the results. The median value is often a better way to describe data. Median refers to the exact middle. 50 percent of the data would be above the median, and 50 percent would be below. Five people are weighed, and the results are as follows: 130 pounds, 175 pounds, 210 pounds, 155 pounds, and 195 pounds. The mean weight would be 173 pounds, and the median weight would be 175 pounds. Mode refers to the value that is seen most often in the data set. Mode is used less often than median and mean.

147. B: A data collection instrument can consist of behavior assessments, interview questions for individuals or groups, focus groups, or surveys. In order for the data collection instrument to be used in research, it must be considered validated and reliable. Existing data collection instruments are available; however, it is time consuming to determine what instruments are available, how to obtain them, and how to locate the author. Some researchers will use certain parts of a preexisting instrument. It is often difficult to locate the author for permission. Some instruments are copyrighted, but the authors are more than willing to share their instruments with other researchers. Some authors will require that the researcher have a certain type of credential, while other authors will require a fee for use of the instrument or that any published data be shared with the author. It is also time consuming and difficult to develop an original data collection instrument, but sometimes this must be the solution if a preexisting instrument is not located.

148. C: Strategic planning involves a process used to identify larger goals and how these will be achieved. The first question that must be answered is "where are we now?" This provides a definitive picture of the current state of affairs. Strengths and weaknesses of the organization are identified as well as any potential barriers or obstacles. Key stakeholders are identified and assessed. The next question involves the direction the organization would like to go. This would also include a time frame to achieving both short- and long-term goals. The third question is

"How do we get to this place to achieve the goals?" An analysis must be conducted of resources, staffing, skills, and required training. Various ways to achieve the goals should be identified. The person in charge of achieving the goals of strategic planning must also be identified.

149. D: Establishing a base of volunteers to help with administering a program can be difficult. People have full-time jobs, family or social obligations, or other commitments that make it difficult to commit to volunteering. Effective recruiting is essential because it will save both time and money if it is done in the appropriate manner. The most effective method of recruiting individuals to volunteer is by personal invitation. If an individual is identified as having a desirable skill set that would help with the program, a friend can contact that individual and try to obtain a commitment. Other ways to recruit can include a media campaign or speaking with individuals who attend community events. An example of this may be going to a walk designated to the cause being promoted and talking to people there. College or high school students are another potential source of volunteers because many schools and programs require service hours. Retirees are another potential source for individuals looking to give back to the community.

150. B: When establishing a training session for potential volunteers, it is important to take into account a variety of schedules and locations to try to meet the majority of needs. If training is offered only once per month, it is inflexible and may not accommodate all potential volunteers. Training that is offered to paid staff can also be opened up to volunteers. It is important to introduce volunteers to the organization, staff, policies, and procedures as well as the mission of the organization. The overall needs of the volunteers should be assessed and addressed. The amount of training required will be dependent in part on this. Supporting the volunteers is also important, as the individuals may have concerns or specific goals in mind for their service commitment. Support should continue throughout the volunteer service process.

151. C: The development of a volunteer's policy and procedure document is a good way to support volunteers as well as to provide consistency to the organization. There are many points that can be addressed in this document, including how volunteers relate to the functioning of the organization and the mission of the organization. It also includes the recruitment policy, issues surrounding diversity and equal opportunity, orientation and training, and support. The document can also cover how volunteers are insured and what is done to protect the health and safety of the volunteers. Confidentiality agreements are often included along with how the organization deals with complaints about volunteers. The handling of any volunteer expenses should also be addressed, specifying what the reimbursement policy is and what it might cover.

152. A: Screening potential volunteers is similar to hiring employees, and many of the same laws apply. It is important to screen volunteers for both the individual's protection as well as the individuals receiving the service. Medical history should not be obtained as well as religious or sexual orientation. Criminal background checks are extremely important, especially if the volunteer will be working with vulnerable groups such as children or the elderly. Driving records can be checked as well. Personal references should be verified and followed up to determine the suitability of the individual to the volunteer position. Risk management strategies should be utilized when conducting the screenings; for example, a potential candidate may not be considered if a certain number of moving violations have been incurred if applying for a volunteer driver position. Written screening guidelines should be developed so the screening process is consistent. Individuals should always provide consent before background checks are conducted.

153. B: When developing health education materials, it is important to use plain language. This helps to ensure that those individuals with lower health literacy are able to understand and process the information being presented. Plain language is a process used to help make written or oral information easier to understand. The information is presented in such a way that it can be understood the first time it is read or heard. The information should be organized so the most important points are presented first, and sentences should be short and concise. Any complicated information or facts are broken into smaller ideas. An active voice is used, and the language selected is simple. The reading level for health-related information should be around a fourth- or fifth-grade reading level.

154. D: There are many databases available for a variety of topics. Databases that specialize in medical literature can be used to access professional journals for research purposes. Medline is part of PubMed and is a free online database of more than 5,400 journals. It is easy to search and find the information that is needed. Cochrane Review is a collaboration of reviews of primary research that has been done involving health and healthcare policy. ERIC, the Educational Resources Information Center, is a large database of education literature. Although this is an invaluable tool, it would not be helpful in a medical literature search.

155. C: Healthfinder.gov is a government Web site that has information pertaining to a large number of health topics. It includes health tools, links to information on other Web sites, and assistance with finding additional services or information. It utilizes other government Web sites as well as nonprofit organizations that provide reliable and trustworthy medical information. This Web site does not accept any paid advertising. It would be a good Web site to refer program participants to if additional information was needed on a particular topic. For example, if a participant attended a program dealing with Type 2 diabetes, they would be able to find additional Web sites with good information, including the American Diabetes Association, the National Diabetes Education Program, and the National Institutes of Health. The participant would still have to do a search, but using this Web site would ensure that reliable Web sites are selected.

156. C: The main difference between an internal consultant and an external consultant is a contract. An external consultant works with outside clients and provides more technical type information and is often process oriented. A contract is usually written to specify exactly what services will be provided by an external consultant. An internal consultant often works informally by advising colleagues and will act as a resource person on regarding certain issues. Both internal and external consultants require specialized knowledge and are expected to remain current with recent theories and research. A consultant's role is to help develop a plan of action based on the needs of the client or colleague.

157. A: Each of the listed groups would certainly be important parts of a task force addressing underage drinking. The inclusion of the target population (in this case teenagers or high school students) would be extremely important. Research has shown that peer educators are an important resource in any topic. Peer educators can help shape and influence behaviors and help to build relationships between teachers and students or teachers and law enforcement. It is important to adequately train peer educators and to help address logistical issues that may arise such as schedules or transportation to meetings. Students willing to be peer educators will gain leadership and other skills such as public speaking.

158. D: Identifying the priority population is an important step in the providing the most effective health education program. There are significant amounts of data available to identify the populations that should be targeted for antismoking efforts. These populations would include ethnicity of American Indians, Alaskan natives, and African Americans. Those with income levels that are around the poverty level would also be good targets for an antismoking campaign. Priority populations could also include those with less than a high school education or a GED. If the population was to be identified by geographic location, the Midwest or the Southeast would be the best areas to target, as these two regions have the highest rates of adult smoking.

159. A: The Coalition of National Health Education Organizations published its revised Code of Ethics for the Health Education Profession in February of 2011. This document is designed to provide guidance in decision-making and behavior by any health educator. There are six articles that are covered. These include responsibility to the public, responsibility to the profession, responsibility to employers, responsibility in the delivery of health education, responsibility in research and evaluation, and responsibility in professional preparation. The ethical principles that govern the code are to promote justice, doing good, and doing no harm, which is similar to other areas of health care, such as those for physicians. Diversity and cultural awareness are also part of the code. The code can be read in full at http://www.cnheo.org/.

160. C: Healthy People 2020 is a 10-year national plan for improving the health and well-being of all Americans. The program is managed by the United States Department of Health and Human Services and has been in existence for more than 30 years. Healthy People 2020 covers many topics, and 13 new topics were introduced with the latest revision, including adolescent health, early and middle childhood, older adults, sleep health, health care associated infections, global health, and dementia. Previous topics include information on many disease states such as cancer, chronic kidney disease, HIV, arthritis, weight, and heart disease. It is an excellent tool for a health educator to utilize for guidance and resources for a variety of health-related issues. There is information for consumers, community-based interventions, and clinical interventions. The Web site for Healthy People 2020 is http://www.healthypeople.gov/.

161. B: One of the skills required of health educators is networking. This involves meeting other professionals and establishing a relationship with these people. Maintaining contact is important, so when an issue arises that requires outside assistance, a list of professionals willing to help or give an opinion is readily available. A health educator is not expected to know everything there is to know about health. What is important is knowing how to get the information needed. Networking contacts may include physicians, other nurses, dentists, registered dietitians, other health educators, pharmacists, or any other type of healthcare professional. A list of contacts obtained through networking takes time and effort to obtain.

162. A: A lay health education specialist is someone who has been extensively trained to provide a certain type of health education. Typically, the lay health education specialist is trained by a certified health education specialist (CHES) or another healthcare provider. The lay health education specialist can be someone in the community who would be able to make an impact on educating a certain population such as a youth pastor providing education about sexually transmitted diseases or drug abuse to at-risk teens in the church community. These lay health education specialists can also help to lobby various government agencies when needed and would be able to knowledgably present the information. They are also referred to as community health advisors or advocates. To be a CHES or certified health education specialist, certain academic qualifications must be established first, and most lay health education specialist will not qualify to sit for the national exam

163. D: Literacy levels are a major barrier to delivering health education as well as to individuals understanding the information being provided. Populations with a high number of individuals with either basic or below-basic literacy levels typically have poorer health. Because of this, healthcare costs are higher. Areas with low literacy also tend to have populations with less education and lower incomes. Access to technology such as the Internet is less prevalent. Those with low literacy are less able to look at health messages being delivered by the media and evaluate what they see or hear. As many as 20% of all adults do not have adequate literacy skills. It is important to address this when planning health education by using simple materials that incorporate a variety of graphics as well as examples to illustrate points. The amount of white space on a page needs to be balanced with the number of words. The reading level should be kept to around a fourth- or fifth-grade level.

164. A: Sending a letter through the mail to any legislator requires a bioterrorism screening before it can reach the office. Using a form letter is less effective. Many legislators would prefer a handwritten letter that shows someone took the actual time to sit and write it. A faxed letter will be received more quickly. Care should be taken to properly address any letter that is sent to a legislator. Email is another good way and can be effective if it is not sent in a blanket mailing but is rather addressed specifically to the state representative that is being contacted. A telephone call is always effective, as is making an appointment for a personal visit.

165. C: Every health education specialist, like most professionals working in health care, need to make a plan for personal and professional growth. In order to maintain CHES certification, 75 continuing education contact hours must be obtained every 5 years. There are many ways to maintain and plan for growth, including reading professional journals, attending interesting professional meetings or seminars, or taking courses at a local university. These may also include writing a professional journal article or a chapter in a book. Many individuals find enjoyment in presenting at local or national professional meetings. Obtaining an appropriate master's degree is another route to professional growth. It is also important to stay current with technology, as it changes rapidly. This includes social media, various types of software such as PowerPoint or word processing, Internet search engines and techniques for searching, and developing Web pages.

How to Overcome Test Anxiety

Just the thought of taking a test is enough to make most people a little nervous. A test is an important event that can have a long-term impact on your future, so it's important to take it seriously and it's natural to feel anxious about performing well. But just because anxiety is normal, that doesn't mean that it's helpful in test taking, or that you should simply accept it as part of your life. Anxiety can have a variety of effects. These effects can be mild, like making you feel slightly nervous, or severe, like blocking your ability to focus or remember even a simple detail.

If you experience test anxiety—whether severe or mild—it's important to know how to beat it. To discover this, first you need to understand what causes test anxiety.

Causes of Test Anxiety

While we often think of anxiety as an uncontrollable emotional state, it can actually be caused by simple, practical things. One of the most common causes of test anxiety is that a person does not feel adequately prepared for their test. This feeling can be the result of many different issues such as poor study habits or lack of organization, but the most common culprit is time management. Starting to study too late, failing to organize your study time to cover all of the material, or being distracted while you study will mean that you're not well prepared for the test. This may lead to cramming the night before, which will cause you to be physically and mentally exhausted for the test. Poor time management also contributes to feelings of stress, fear, and hopelessness as you realize you are not well prepared but don't know what to do about it.

Other times, test anxiety is not related to your preparation for the test but comes from unresolved fear. This may be a past failure on a test, or poor performance on tests in general. It may come from comparing yourself to others who seem to be performing better or from the stress of living up to expectations. Anxiety may be driven by fears of the future—how failure on this test would affect your educational and career goals. These fears are often completely irrational, but they can still negatively impact your test performance.

> **Review Video: 3 Reasons You Have Test Anxiety**
> Visit mometrix.com/academy and enter code: 428468

155

Elements of Test Anxiety

As mentioned earlier, test anxiety is considered to be an emotional state, but it has physical and mental components as well. Sometimes you may not even realize that you are suffering from test anxiety until you notice the physical symptoms. These can include trembling hands, rapid heartbeat, sweating, nausea, and tense muscles. Extreme anxiety may lead to fainting or vomiting. Obviously, any of these symptoms can have a negative impact on testing. It is important to recognize them as soon as they begin to occur so that you can address the problem before it damages your performance.

Review Video: 3 Ways to Tell You Have Test Anxiety
Visit mometrix.com/academy and enter code: 927847

The mental components of test anxiety include trouble focusing and inability to remember learned information. During a test, your mind is on high alert, which can help you recall information and stay focused for an extended period of time. However, anxiety interferes with your mind's natural processes, causing you to blank out, even on the questions you know well. The strain of testing during anxiety makes it difficult to stay focused, especially on a test that may take several hours. Extreme anxiety can take a huge mental toll, making it difficult not only to recall test information but even to understand the test questions or pull your thoughts together.

Review Video: How Test Anxiety Affects Memory
Visit mometrix.com/academy and enter code: 609003

Effects of Test Anxiety

Test anxiety is like a disease—if left untreated, it will get progressively worse. Anxiety leads to poor performance, and this reinforces the feelings of fear and failure, which in turn lead to poor performances on subsequent tests. It can grow from a mild nervousness to a crippling condition. If allowed to progress, test anxiety can have a big impact on your schooling, and consequently on your future.

Test anxiety can spread to other parts of your life. Anxiety on tests can become anxiety in any stressful situation, and blanking on a test can turn into panicking in a job situation. But fortunately, you don't have to let anxiety rule your testing and determine your grades. There are a number of relatively simple steps you can take to move past anxiety and function normally on a test and in the rest of life.

Review Video: How Test Anxiety Impacts Your Grades
Visit mometrix.com/academy and enter code: 939819

Physical Steps for Beating Test Anxiety

While test anxiety is a serious problem, the good news is that it can be overcome. It doesn't have to control your ability to think and remember information. While it may take time, you can begin taking steps today to beat anxiety.

Just as your first hint that you may be struggling with anxiety comes from the physical symptoms, the first step to treating it is also physical. Rest is crucial for having a clear, strong mind. If you are tired, it is much easier to give in to anxiety. But if you establish good sleep habits, your body and mind will be ready to perform optimally, without the strain of exhaustion. Additionally, sleeping well helps you to retain information better, so you're more likely to recall the answers when you see the test questions.

Getting good sleep means more than going to bed on time. It's important to allow your brain time to relax. Take study breaks from time to time so it doesn't get overworked, and don't study right before bed. Take time to rest your mind before trying to rest your body, or you may find it difficult to fall asleep.

> **Review Video: The Importance of Sleep for Your Brain**
> Visit mometrix.com/academy and enter code: 319338

Along with sleep, other aspects of physical health are important in preparing for a test. Good nutrition is vital for good brain function. Sugary foods and drinks may give a burst of energy but this burst is followed by a crash, both physically and emotionally. Instead, fuel your body with protein and vitamin-rich foods.

Also, drink plenty of water. Dehydration can lead to headaches and exhaustion, especially if your brain is already under stress from the rigors of the test. Particularly if your test is a long one, drink water during the breaks. And if possible, take an energy-boosting snack to eat between sections.

> **Review Video: How Diet Can Affect your Mood**
> Visit mometrix.com/academy and enter code: 624317

Along with sleep and diet, a third important part of physical health is exercise. Maintaining a steady workout schedule is helpful, but even taking 5-minute study breaks to walk can help get your blood pumping faster and clear your head. Exercise also releases endorphins, which contribute to a positive feeling and can help combat test anxiety.

When you nurture your physical health, you are also contributing to your mental health. If your body is healthy, your mind is much more likely to be healthy as well. So take time to rest, nourish your body with healthy food and water, and get moving as much as possible. Taking these physical steps will make you stronger and more able to take the mental steps necessary to overcome test anxiety.

> **Review Video: How to Stay Healthy and Prevent Test Anxiety**
> Visit mometrix.com/academy and enter code: 877894

Mental Steps for Beating Test Anxiety

Working on the mental side of test anxiety can be more challenging, but as with the physical side, there are clear steps you can take to overcome it. As mentioned earlier, test anxiety often stems from lack of preparation, so the obvious solution is to prepare for the test. Effective studying may be the most important weapon you have for beating test anxiety, but you can and should employ several other mental tools to combat fear.

First, boost your confidence by reminding yourself of past success—tests or projects that you aced. If you're putting as much effort into preparing for this test as you did for those, there's no reason you should expect to fail here. Work hard to prepare; then trust your preparation.

Second, surround yourself with encouraging people. It can be helpful to find a study group, but be sure that the people you're around will encourage a positive attitude. If you spend time with others who are anxious or cynical, this will only contribute to your own anxiety. Look for others who are motivated to study hard from a desire to succeed, not from a fear of failure.

Third, reward yourself. A test is physically and mentally tiring, even without anxiety, and it can be helpful to have something to look forward to. Plan an activity following the test, regardless of the outcome, such as going to a movie or getting ice cream.

When you are taking the test, if you find yourself beginning to feel anxious, remind yourself that you know the material. Visualize successfully completing the test. Then take a few deep, relaxing breaths and return to it. Work through the questions carefully but with confidence, knowing that you are capable of succeeding.

Developing a healthy mental approach to test taking will also aid in other areas of life. Test anxiety affects more than just the actual test—it can be damaging to your mental health and even contribute to depression. It's important to beat test anxiety before it becomes a problem for more than testing.

Review Video: Test Anxiety and Depression
Visit mometrix.com/academy and enter code: 904704

Study Strategy

Being prepared for the test is necessary to combat anxiety, but what does being prepared look like? You may study for hours on end and still not feel prepared. What you need is a strategy for test prep. The next few pages outline our recommended steps to help you plan out and conquer the challenge of preparation.

STEP 1: SCOPE OUT THE TEST

Learn everything you can about the format (multiple choice, essay, etc.) and what will be on the test. Gather any study materials, course outlines, or sample exams that may be available. Not only will this help you to prepare, but knowing what to expect can help to alleviate test anxiety.

STEP 2: MAP OUT THE MATERIAL

Look through the textbook or study guide and make note of how many chapters or sections it has. Then divide these over the time you have. For example, if a book has 15 chapters and you have five days to study, you need to cover three chapters each day. Even better, if you have the time, leave an extra day at the end for overall review after you have gone through the material in depth.

If time is limited, you may need to prioritize the material. Look through it and make note of which sections you think you already have a good grasp on, and which need review. While you are studying, skim quickly through the familiar sections and take more time on the challenging parts. Write out your plan so you don't get lost as you go. Having a written plan also helps you feel more in control of the study, so anxiety is less likely to arise from feeling overwhelmed at the amount to cover. A sample plan may look like this:

- Day 1: Skim chapters 1–4, study chapter 5 (especially pages 31–33)
- Day 2: Study chapters 6–7, skim chapters 8–9
- Day 3: Skim chapter 10, study chapters 11–12 (especially pages 87–90)
- Day 4: Study chapters 13–15
- Day 5: Overall review (focus most on chapters 5, 6, and 12), take practice test

STEP 3: GATHER YOUR TOOLS

Decide what study method works best for you. Do you prefer to highlight in the book as you study and then go back over the highlighted portions? Or do you type out notes of the important information? Or is it helpful to make flashcards that you can carry with you? Assemble the pens, index cards, highlighters, post-it notes, and any other materials you may need so you won't be distracted by getting up to find things while you study.

If you're having a hard time retaining the information or organizing your notes, experiment with different methods. For example, try color-coding by subject with colored pens, highlighters, or post-it notes. If you learn better by hearing, try recording yourself reading your notes so you can listen while in the car, working out, or simply sitting at your desk. Ask a friend to quiz you from your flashcards, or try teaching someone the material to solidify it in your mind.

STEP 4: CREATE YOUR ENVIRONMENT

It's important to avoid distractions while you study. This includes both the obvious distractions like visitors and the subtle distractions like an uncomfortable chair (or a too-comfortable couch that makes you want to fall asleep). Set up the best study environment possible: good lighting and a comfortable work area. If background music helps you focus, you may want to turn it on, but otherwise keep the room quiet. If you are using a computer to take notes, be sure you don't have any other windows open, especially applications like social media, games, or anything else that could distract you. Silence your phone and turn off notifications. Be sure to keep water close by so you stay hydrated while you study (but avoid unhealthy drinks and snacks).

Also, take into account the best time of day to study. Are you freshest first thing in the morning? Try to set aside some time then to work through the material. Is your mind clearer in the afternoon or evening? Schedule your study session then. Another method is to study at the same time of day that you will take the test, so that your brain gets used to working on the material at that time and will be ready to focus at test time.

STEP 5: STUDY!

Once you have done all the study preparation, it's time to settle into the actual studying. Sit down, take a few moments to settle your mind so you can focus, and begin to follow your study plan. Don't give in to distractions or let yourself procrastinate. This is your time to prepare so you'll be ready to fearlessly approach the test. Make the most of the time and stay focused.

Of course, you don't want to burn out. If you study too long you may find that you're not retaining the information very well. Take regular study breaks. For example, taking five minutes out of every hour to walk briskly, breathing deeply and swinging your arms, can help your mind stay fresh.

As you get to the end of each chapter or section, it's a good idea to do a quick review. Remind yourself of what you learned and work on any difficult parts. When you feel that you've mastered the material, move on to the next part. At the end of your study session, briefly skim through your notes again.

But while review is helpful, cramming last minute is NOT. If at all possible, work ahead so that you won't need to fit all your study into the last day. Cramming overloads your brain with more information than it can process and retain, and your tired mind may struggle to recall even previously learned information when it is overwhelmed with last-minute study. Also, the urgent nature of cramming and the stress placed on your brain contribute to anxiety. You'll be more likely to go to the test feeling unprepared and having trouble thinking clearly.

So don't cram, and don't stay up late before the test, even just to review your notes at a leisurely pace. Your brain needs rest more than it needs to go over the information again. In fact, plan to finish your studies by noon or early afternoon the day before the test. Give your brain the rest of the day to relax or focus on other things, and get a good night's sleep. Then you will be fresh for the test and better able to recall what you've studied.

STEP 6: TAKE A PRACTICE TEST

Many courses offer sample tests, either online or in the study materials. This is an excellent resource to check whether you have mastered the material, as well as to prepare for the test format and environment.

Check the test format ahead of time: the number of questions, the type (multiple choice, free response, etc.), and the time limit. Then create a plan for working through them. For example, if you have 30 minutes to take a 60-question test, your limit is 30 seconds per question. Spend less time on the questions you know well so that you can take more time on the difficult ones.

If you have time to take several practice tests, take the first one open book, with no time limit. Work through the questions at your own pace and make sure you fully understand them. Gradually work up to taking a test under test conditions: sit at a desk with all study materials put away and set a timer. Pace yourself to make sure you finish the test with time to spare and go back to check your answers if you have time.

After each test, check your answers. On the questions you missed, be sure you understand why you missed them. Did you misread the question (tests can use tricky wording)? Did you forget the information? Or was it something you hadn't learned? Go back and study any shaky areas that the practice tests reveal.

Taking these tests not only helps with your grade, but also aids in combating test anxiety. If you're already used to the test conditions, you're less likely to worry about it, and working through tests until you're scoring well gives you a confidence boost. Go through the practice tests until you feel comfortable, and then you can go into the test knowing that you're ready for it.

Test Tips

On test day, you should be confident, knowing that you've prepared well and are ready to answer the questions. But aside from preparation, there are several test day strategies you can employ to maximize your performance.

First, as stated before, get a good night's sleep the night before the test (and for several nights before that, if possible). Go into the test with a fresh, alert mind rather than staying up late to study.

Try not to change too much about your normal routine on the day of the test. It's important to eat a nutritious breakfast, but if you normally don't eat breakfast at all, consider eating just a protein bar. If you're a coffee drinker, go ahead and have your normal coffee. Just make sure you time it so that the caffeine doesn't wear off right in the middle of your test. Avoid sugary beverages, and drink enough water to stay hydrated but not so much that you need a restroom break 10 minutes into the test. If your test isn't first thing in the morning, consider going for a walk or doing a light workout before the test to get your blood flowing.

Allow yourself enough time to get ready, and leave for the test with plenty of time to spare so you won't have the anxiety of scrambling to arrive in time. Another reason to be early is to select a good seat. It's helpful to sit away from doors and windows, which can be distracting. Find a good seat, get out your supplies, and settle your mind before the test begins.

When the test begins, start by going over the instructions carefully, even if you already know what to expect. Make sure you avoid any careless mistakes by following the directions.

Then begin working through the questions, pacing yourself as you've practiced. If you're not sure on an answer, don't spend too much time on it, and don't let it shake your confidence. Either skip it and come back later, or eliminate as many wrong answers as possible and guess among the remaining ones. Don't dwell on these questions as you continue—put them out of your mind and focus on what lies ahead.

Be sure to read all of the answer choices, even if you're sure the first one is the right answer. Sometimes you'll find a better one if you keep reading. But don't second-guess yourself if you do immediately know the answer. Your gut instinct is usually right. Don't let test anxiety rob you of the information you know.

If you have time at the end of the test (and if the test format allows), go back and review your answers. Be cautious about changing any, since your first instinct tends to be correct, but make sure you didn't misread any of the questions or accidentally mark the wrong answer choice. Look over any you skipped and make an educated guess.

At the end, leave the test feeling confident. You've done your best, so don't waste time worrying about your performance or wishing you could change anything. Instead, celebrate the successful completion of this test. And finally, use this test to learn how to deal with anxiety even better next time.

Review Video: 5 Tips to Beat Test Anxiety
Visit mometrix.com/academy and enter code: 570656

Important Qualification

Not all anxiety is created equal. If your test anxiety is causing major issues in your life beyond the classroom or testing center, or if you are experiencing troubling physical symptoms related to your anxiety, it may be a sign of a serious physiological or psychological condition. If this sounds like your situation, we strongly encourage you to seek professional help.

Thank You

We at Mometrix would like to extend our heartfelt thanks to you, our friend and patron, for allowing us to play a part in your journey. It is a privilege to serve people from all walks of life who are unified in their commitment to building the best future they can for themselves.

The preparation you devote to these important testing milestones may be the most valuable educational opportunity you have for making a real difference in your life. We encourage you to put your heart into it—that feeling of succeeding, overcoming, and yes, conquering will be well worth the hours you've invested.

We want to hear your story, your struggles and your successes, and if you see any opportunities for us to improve our materials so we can help others even more effectively in the future, please share that with us as well. **The team at Mometrix would be absolutely thrilled to hear from you!** So please, send us an email (support@mometrix.com) and let's stay in touch.

> **If you'd like some additional help, check out these other resources we offer for your exam:**
> **http://MometrixFlashcards.com/CHES**

Additional Bonus Material

Due to our efforts to try to keep this book to a manageable length, we've created a link that will give you access to all of your additional bonus material.

Please visit http://www.mometrix.com/bonus948/ches to access the information.